Reproductive Clinical Problems in the Dog

A Veterinary Practitioner Handbook
Series Edited by Neal King BVSC MRCVS

REPRODUCTIVE CLINICAL PROBLEMS IN THE DOG

D. Edward Jones BSc, BVSc, PhD, MRCVS
Lecturer in Veterinary Clinical Studies (Small Animals)
University of Liverpool

Joan O. Joshua FRCVS
formerly Reader in Veterinary Surgery (Small Animals)
University of Liverpool

WRIGHT·PSG

Bristol London Boston
1982

Published by:
John Wright & Sons Ltd, 42–44 Triangle West, Bristol BS8 1EX, England

John Wright PSG Inc.,
545 Great Road, Littleton, Massachusetts 01460, USA.

British Library Cataloguing in Publication Data
Joshua, Joan O.
 Reproductive clinical problems in the
 dog. – (A Veterinary practitioner
 handbook)
 1. Dogs–Reproduction
 I. Title II. Jones, D. Edward   III. Series
 636.7′0824   SF991

ISBN 0 7236 0638 2
Library of Congress Catalog Card Number: 81-70757

Typeset by Activity, Salisbury, Wiltshire
and printed in Great Britain by
John Wright & Sons (Printing) Ltd., at the Stonebridge Press, Bristol, BS4 5NU

Preface

The controlled breeding, by man, of many subspecies has been in progress for so long that the numerous established, domesticated varieties are now more universally familiar than their forebears. Yet concepts of breeding control are generally alien to the layman, except in the context of the companion animals with which he is most closely associated, and even within that context he is mostly unaware that greater extremes of manipulative coupling are indulged by the goldfish breeder than are contemplated by dog- or cat-breeding fraternities.

Due to this lack of awareness a disproportionate amount of attention is now paid by the lay press, and to some extent by the small-animal veterinary press, to the activities of the dog breeder and his veterinary surgeon.

Both authors, as veterinary clinicians who are also dog breeders and exhibitors, are thoroughly conversant with the aspirations of the dog breeder, the sometimes problematical role of his veterinary surgeon and, by no means least, with the requirements of and problems faced by the pet-owning public into whose homes the majority of puppies are eventually placed. D. Edward Jones, having most experience of sight hounds in which major problems are assumed not to occur, has, nevertheless, been interested to observe disease trends of relatively minor significance apparent within particular bloodlines and breeding patterns. Joan Joshua, having a half-century's experience of breeding and exhibiting that true fancier variety, the Chow, is familiar at first hand with the need for common sense and integrity in the useful application of breed knowledge for the production of sound stock in a problematical breed.

Both authors regard dog breeding as an absorbing hobby ethically compatible with broad humanitarian principles, but recognize a distinction between the possible and the permissible in the context of veterinary assistance to the dog breeder. It is with this distinction in mind that several procedures are discussed which may be argued, by their uncontrolled practice, to exceed the bounds of ethical veterinary practice either because of their detriment to the individual animal or to the breed in general. When appropriate, the ethical stance of the authors will be stated.

February
1982

D.E.J.
J.O.J.

Contents

Chapter 1

Ovary, Fallopian Tubes and Associated Structures

OVARY, OVARIAN LIGAMENTS AND FAT BURSA

Anatomical features of clinical significance

Ovaries
The ovaries of the bitch are paired oval organs derived embryologically from the ventromedial portion of the intermediate cell mass and located, after some caudal migration, suspended in the broad ligaments within the abdominal cavity caudal to the kidneys. The precise location varies and the ovaries are more caudally and ventrally placed in bitches which have undergone several pregnancies.

Ovaries are relatively small, approximately 1·5 x 0·7 x 0·5 cm in a 25-lb bitch, and smooth-surfaced, although after several oestrous cycles, and particularly following pregnancies, the surface is noticeably rough and nodular. Blood supply is by ovarian arteries and by anastomosis from uterine arteries. Venous drainage is into the posterior vena cava and renal veins and by anastomosis into uterine veins.

Each ovary comprises a central medulla of supporting vascularity, etc. and an outer cortex containing within its connective tissue stroma, numerous germ cells and follicles in various stages of development according to the phase of oestrous cyclic activity.

There are two features of the canine ovary which are very relevant to veterinary practice and especially surgery; these are the shortness and conformation of the ovarian ligament and the well-developed fat bursa which encloses the ovary.

Ovarian ligament
This is not only short but tends to be fan-shaped which makes the laying

1

of ligatures below the ovary difficult and predisposes to slipping of the ligature.

The suspensory ligament which attaches the ovary cranially is short, tense and tough but it is also relatively avascular. It is this ligament which makes access to the ovary, whether by the midline or flank approach, so difficult in the bitch. However, as it is free of large blood vessels it can be safely severed at the cranial edge by blunt or sharp dissection and the remainder of the ligament can be separated carefully until the large vessels, the anastomosis of the uterine and ovarian vessels near the cranial extremity of the uterine horns, are reached. Ligatures can then be securely and precisely applied. Since the main blood flow is retrograde from the uterine vessels it is these which must be carefully ligatured in any surgery of the area. The ovarian vessels should also be ligated but all small-animal surgeons will admit that even if this is not achieved, haemorrhage is seldom serious.

Fat bursa

This is particularly well developed in the bitch and is present from quite an early age; it also persists even in emaciated subjects for longer than most other body fat. The fat bursa effectively masks the ovary itself which can only be seen in its entirety when it is extruded from the bursa. For this reason it is vital in all surgical procedures involving ovariectomy that the genital tract removed should be carefully examined to ensure that no ovarian tissue has been left in situ. As all clinicians know, cases of oestrous cycles persisting after alleged ovariectomy arise from time to time and can be a cause of anxiety to surgeon and owner alike.

Physiological features of the ovary

Derived from the germinal layer of ovarian epithelium by ingrowth, probably during fetal life, are cords of germ cells which produce ova-bearing follicles. Although many of these degenerate and become atretic, others, the Graafian follicles, develop in response to hormonally governed cyclic ovarian activity. After migration to the serosa-free surface of the ovary they rupture, shedding ova into the ovarian bursa. Each follicle, after shedding its ovum, matures to become a hormone-producing corpus luteum before finally degenerating into connective scar tissue.

The cyclic sexual patterns of the bitch are distinctively different from those of other domesticated species and will be discussed in detail in Chapter 4. Although debate continues over minutiae, it is generally agreed that the bitch be termed seasonally monocyclic, having only one crop of follicles mature at each 'season' or 'heat', these seasons being separated by prolonged periods of apparent sexual quiescence. Despite its differences, however, for practical purposes the bitch ovary may be assumed, as in other species, to be controlled by the pituitary release of gonadotrophins, and to be susceptible to the interplay between these and the hormones of the ovarian and other organs.

What is most remarkable in the bitch is the post-ovulatory phase of follicular change with development of full luteal function even in the absence of pregnancy. A range of physiological and pathological changes which are not commonly encountered in other domesticated species are attributable to this.

Pathological conditions of the ovary

Tumours

Ovarian tumours are not uncommon and the various types encountered are well documented. They may or may not be hormonally active. Their size is variable, from lesions not recognizable macroscopically to large space-occupying masses which may cause obvious abdominal distension. Hormonally active tumours may cause any one of, or a combination of, the following signs:

> Irregularity of oestrous cycles
> Persistent haemorrhage
> Suppression of cycles
> Nymphomania
> Hair loss usually seen as a bilaterally symmetrical alopecia
> of the upper flank area.

Large tumours, which are often not hormonally active, may be un-recognized for a considerable time but will eventually give rise to signs suggestive of a mild obstructive condition, e.g. discomfort on lying, some inappetence and occasionally vomiting. Many remain asymptomatic until abdominal distension is evident or the mass is found during routine abdominal palpation. In general it can be said that a large abdominal mass which is not causing signs clearly related to another organ is likely to be splenic or ovarian in origin. Treatment is by surgical removal of the ovary(ies), which is usually a reasonably routine procedure.

Nymphomania

This term is not entirely accurate as affected bitches do not necessarily show increased libido. Clinically three syndromes are recognizable.

1. Irregular and frequent cycles which are not fully developed seasons, e.g. the vulva may show a degree of swelling which can even vary from day to day. Attraction to males is variable as is the bitch's willingness to accept service. Quiescent periods are brief and difficult to identify, i.e. the bitch may not appear to be oestrous but is nonetheless pestered by dogs. Vaginal discharge may or may not be present.

2. Bitches which show a persistent desire to escape even though physical changes in the external genitalia are not recognizable. These bitches are often pestered by dogs and may even be apparently 'raped'.

3. Bitches in which bleeding and vulvovaginal swelling persist for considerable periods of time and sometimes appear to indicate abnormal prolongation of heat cycle.

In all these cases the ovaries are likely to show the following changes: the presence of numerous thin-walled Graafian follicles (occasionally macroscopically recognizable and causing enlargement of the ovarian bursa) with little evidence of corpora lutea. The uterus shows changes in the endometrium.

Clinically the important feature is that response to medical treatment is usually disappointing and ovariectomy is the procedure of choice. In view of the endometrial changes which may be present it is prudent to remove the uterus; in any case the uterus is of no further use to an ovariectomized bitch.

OVIDUCTS (Fallopian Tubes)

These also are largely concealed in the fat bursa and their recognition is difficult during quiescent phases of the reproductive cycle; hence exploratory laparatomy in cases of infertility is not always a rewarding procedure.

Very little attention has been paid to this vital section of the reproductive tract although Miller et al. (1964) state that congenital stenosis of the oviduct is not infrequent. The authors have on record the case of one non-breeding chow bitch which at postmortem examination was found to have no oviducts, their site being merely represented by fibrous strands. Thus congenital agenesis of the oviducts can occur. Whether adhesions within the oviducts can arise following bacterial infection of the genital tract is speculative, and procedures to establish patency or otherwise are seldom undertaken.

REFERENCE

Miller M. E., Christensen G. C. and Evans H. E. (1964). *Anatomy of the Dog.* W. B. Saunders Co., Philadelphia: London.

Chapter 2

Uterus and Cervix

APPLIED ANATOMY AND PHYSIOLOGY OF UTERUS

The horns of the muscular, bicornuate uterus extend backwards from their Fallopian tube connections in the region of the kidneys to a prepelvic point of convergence where they unite to form a single short tube, the body or fundus, inserted between the bladder and rectum (*Fig.* 1). The horns are suspended in peritoneal folds — the broad ligaments — carrying in their free edges feeble, fibrous cords — the round ligaments — running

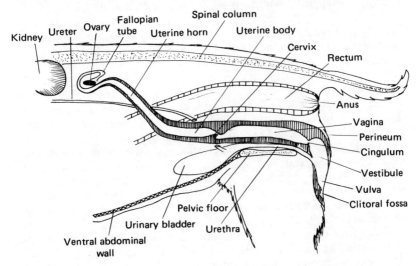

Fig. 1. Sagittal section of bitch to show normal genital canal and its relationship to major organs.

5

back through the inguinal canals to points of insertion in the vulval region. Anterior uterine blood supply is from branches of the utero-ovarian artery running back to anastomose with the posterior supply which derives from the uterine artery, arising from the visceral part of the internal iliac artery and ramifying in the body and neck of the uterus and the vagina. The broad ligaments, being relatively avascular, can safely be torn during surgery although in obese subjects problems may be encountered because of their friability and fairly copious venous drainage.

The serosal surface of the uterine body and horns presents a differing appearance according to the maturity of the animal and her individual cyclic habit (*see* Chapter 4). In the prepubertal and anoestrous, nulliparous bitch the surface is smooth; in parous animals and some nulliparous subjects which have experienced recurrent episodes of false pregnancy, the surface presents a longitudinally fissured and wrinkled appearance.

The mucous membrane lining of the horns and body is also longitudinally folded and the cavity of the uterus is small, being particularly constricted at its point of passage to the vagina by the canal of the cervix. In the prepubertal animal and during true anoestrus the membrane is shallow with a low cuboidal epithelium and poorly developed glands and crypts, although in the sexually mature animal a state of almost continuous epithelial change exists, even during periods of apparent sexual quiescence. To some extent comparable changes can be simultaneously observed throughout the entire mucosal lining of the horns, body and cervix, but at some sites, in particular the apparently predetermined zones of placentation, these changes are very much accentuated.

Such endometrial changes as occur are a reflection of fluctuation in the plasma levels of oestrogen and progesterone hormones emanating from cyclic ovarian activity, and may be grossly envisaged as cycles of endometrial exfoliation, or sloughing, followed by regrowth. This process of exfoliation, commencing a few weeks postpartum, or in non-pregnancy some 90 days post-oestrus, is completed within 50 to 55 days, being less total and more rapidly repaired in the non-pregnant animal, but nevertheless extending the effective metoestrous period to approximately 4-5 months to be followed by only a relatively short, true anoestrus prior to the commencement of further cyclic activity.

Clinical and experimental observations confirm that endometrial development and regression are particularly sensitive to progesterone hormone levels in circulation. The tendency of individuals to exhibit relatively gross symptoms of false pregnancy during metoestrus and the high incidence of uterine mucosal disease in the bitch are manifestations of this sensitivity. Histopathological examination of ovaries and uteri obtained from individuals exhibiting symptoms of false pregnancy reveals that in many endometrial changes are confined to hyperplasia in placenta-like zones, with production of milky fluid within the uterine lumen and the presence of active ovarian corpora lutea. In others corpora lutea are absent, and the endometrial changes of varying degrees of severity are totally dissimilar and are more suggestive of oestrogen than progesterone domination.

There is evidence that while the latter may be associated with pituitary malfunction, the former may be properly considered as an intense manifestation of metoestrus within normal limits. Support for this interpretation is provided by the occasional discovery of individuals in late metoestrus or anoestrus in which a unicornuate uterine obstruction has resulted in distension of one horn with accumulated mucoid fluid while the other horn, although itself recently active, has regressed to present a normal endometrial surface and an empty lumen.

The point at which recurrent mucometra and hyperplastic endometrial changes may be regarded as pathological is debatable, but it has been clearly established, most notably in experiments by Dow (1957, 1958, 1959a, b) that gross and pathological changes in the nature and secretory pattern of the endometrium can be induced by adjustment of the prevailing hormonal environment in a manner analogous to that occurring naturally due to cyclic ovarian activity.

It is generally accepted on this basis that naturally occurring endometrial pathology and pyometra is of hormonal aetiology with bacterial infection sometimes present as a secondary complicating factor. It is hypothesized that bacteria of urogenital origin gain entry to the uterus during oestrus and proliferate during metoestrus during the phase of progesterone domination when uterine resistance to infection is minimal.

A great diversity of bacterial species has been isolated from cases of pyometritis. None of these appears to have any particular significance, although it has been suggested that *Escherichia coli*, a common contaminant, may be associated with a wider range of toxic symptoms than other species.

PYOMETRA

Although pyometra is one of the commonest diseases of the bitch reproductive system, most clinicians would agree that it is a condition which still presents problems in practice. Open cases and those which present with a combination of the classical signs are straightforward enough but, since early recognition and prompt treatment are vital to a favourable outcome, it is the atypical cases which cause anxiety.

Age incidence

At one time pyometra was regarded as essentially a disease of the older nulliparous bitch, hence the advice so often quoted that all bitches should be allowed to have one litter to prevent uterine disease in later life. The falsity of this concept has long been recognized.

Although pyometra is commoner in middle life and above — these definitions will vary according to the longevity of the breed — it is well recognized that it can and does occur even after the first oestrous cycle; this situation does not accord with the aetiology as described by Dow (1957) and remains something of a puzzle in this respect. It is essential, therefore, that a diagnosis of pyometra should not be rejected because of the youth of the patient.

Breeding history

It is now realized that this has little bearing on the incidence of pyometra and that even bitches which have bred regularly may develop the disease. A history of some abnormality in periodicity and duration of recent oestrous cycles is sometimes obtained. There is also circumstantial evidence to suggest that bitches, and indeed strains, which have a history of uterine inertia at parturition show a high incidence of pyometra.

Although pyometra is probably commoner in nulliparous or infrequent breeders there is little evidence available as to the relative representation of these groups in the canine population, so that by and large the breeding history of an individual is not particularly helpful.

Incidence related to stage of oestrous cycle

It is widely recognized that pyometra usually occurs during metoestrus, the 10- to 42-day period is often quoted. Whilst this is important in the clinical history it cannot be completely relied upon. Clinical signs can and do follow oestrus without any evidence of metoestrus supervening, e.g. persistence of vaginal bleeding (*see* p. 10). Cases have also been seen well into what should be the anoestrous phase, e.g. 16 weeks post-oestrus, and in many of these there have been no previous signs to suggest uterine disease.

Clinical signs of pyometra

These include a wide range of symptoms from the classical signs of inappetence, vomiting, thirst and polyuria to the apparently unrelated bizarre evidence of skeletal pain.

Closed cases

The above-mentioned signs of inappetence, vomiting, thirst and polyuria occurring in the metoestrous phase of any 'eligible' bitch should put a diagnosis of pyometra at the top of the list of probabilities. The term 'eligible' has been used in preference to 'entire' because pyometra can and does occur in remnants of uterine body left after alleged spaying; thus the fact that a bitch has been spayed cannot be regarded as 100% proof that she cannot have pyometra. This is regrettable but true.

Polydipsia/polyuria

The very noticeable symptom of polydipsia is apparently a secondary consequence of polyuria, itself the result of secondary impairment of renal function. Several aspects of renal function are susceptible to toxic effects of uterine disease, as will be discussed later (p. 13), and it is sometimes difficult to differentiate between them and to prognosticate on the basis of their likely effects upon the outcome of specifically uterine therapy. The glomerular and tubular diseases which result in polyuria are considered to be consequences of the deposition of immune complexes and are relatively transitory in nature, resolving within approximately 14 days of the removal of the toxic source.

Reduced exercise tolerance

This is often a feature of pyometra, but as many bitches become sluggish in metoestrus anyway it cannot be regarded as highly significant. Temperature rise may or may not be present.

Abdominal distension

This is a variable feature of pyometra, due partly to the degree of distension of the uterus and partly to the abdominal conformation of the patient. Palpation will sometimes detect the enlarged uterus but failure to do so does not rule out the diagnosis; in small bitches rectal investigation with the forelimbs of the bitch raised will sometimes enable the distended organ to be recognized.

The degree of distension with fluid is again extremely variable which accounts for problems in both palpation and radiography. Apart from the cases described under the heading of endometritis there is always marked enlargement of the uterus. In some the amount of retained fluid is considerable in which case the uterus becomes thin-walled, more liable to rupture and more difficult to demonstrate by X-ray; abdominal distension is usually marked. Whilst in most cases the distension of the uterine horns is uniform throughout, in some loculations exist; these can vary in size in the one organ and may easily be confused with a pregnancy of 32 to 40 days' duration. Uteri which remain fairly thick-walled yet contain a fairly large quantity of fluid are more easily palpable and more radio-opaque.

Vulval enlargement

This may be more noticeable in some bitches than would be anticipated in a normal metoestrus, but this is not an invariable sign and the finding of a normal-sized vulva in a pyometra suspect should not be considered to nullify the diagnosis.

Evidence of toxaemia

This will supervene in most cases but again there is considerable variation in the rapidity of onset and degree of severity. Weight loss and depression will follow. Under modern conditions of practice cases which have reached an advanced stage of toxicity should seldom be seen, other than instances in which for some reason or another owners have failed to seek advice at a reasonable, earlier stage.

Less usual signs of pyometra include:

Vaginal haemorrhage

This may be an apparent prolongation of an oestrous cycle although careful history taking will often elicit two significant points: first that the vaginal discharge did become less haemorrhagic for the few days which would indicate oestrus, and then a copious blood discharge, usually more profuse than in pro-oestrus, returned and continued.

Secondly, that the heat period appeared normal but after an interval of 7 to 10 days a copious blood discharge developed. Points of interest in connection with both the above are that clinical signs of ill health are absent or minimal and that at operation these are invariably found to be closed cases with no patency of the cervix, the blood apparently deriving from the cervical and cranial vaginal tissues.

Skeletal pain

It is not possible to be precise about what the presenting signs of skeletal pain will be. Cases have been seen in which the patient is apparently quadriplegic and, if of a disc-prone breed, the condition may at first sight seem to be of disc origin; in other cases polyarthritis may suddenly develop with unwillingness or inability to exercise. Muscle pain without joint involvement may also be seen.

Should history taking reveal that the patient is in metoestrus a diagnosis of pyometra should be considered, even though signs suggestive of that condition are not apparent. It is interesting to note that successful surgery results in complete remission of the skeletal signs suggesting that these are of toxic rather than bacterial invasion origin.

Open cases

This term obviously implies that a vaginal discharge of uterine origin (as distinct from vaginal haemorrhage) is present either continuously or intermittently. Closed cases can become open at any time but the continuously discharging open case rarely becomes a closed one.

The colour of the discharge is very variable, possibly due to the initial bacterial contaminant. The typical pyometra discharge has often been described as café au lait! All variations from cream through brownish shades to frankly haemorrhagic are seen; the consistence is thick and purulent and seldom serous or mucoid although a serosanguineous discharge is present in endometritis. Sometimes at clinical examination no vaginal discharge is seen despite the owner's history; this may be due to flushing of the vestibular area from recent urination, and gentle massage of the perineal vagina will often produce a confirmatory specimen.

As indicated above some open cases discharge intermittently due to closing of the cervical canal as uterine pressure falls, only to reappear after an interval of hours or days as pressure builds up again. Some open cases appear to be so from the outset, the discharge being the reason for the owner seeking advice; the history does not indicate a previously closed phase.

However, some closed cases do become open if the cervix relaxes due to intra-uterine pressure. In most such instances an improvement in general health follows the discharge if this is sufficiently copious, but on rare occasions collapse is associated with the onset of discharge. No explanation of this phenomenon can be offered but experience suggests that prognosis is poor in these circumstances. Relaxation of the cervix prior to the onset of discharge does not as a rule give rise to observable signs but very occasionally the bitch shows discomfort similar to that of late first-stage labour.

Open cases are usually less toxic than the closed type and these are better surgical risks despite the operative hazard of making a section through a contaminated vagina.

It may be difficult to persuade an owner that a closed case which has opened with subsequent symptomatic relief is not permanently cured and that surgical treatment is still required. Permanent recovery rarely occurs in these circumstances, but all clinicians can record the occasional case, in which for some reason operative treatment has not been possible, which apparently responds to medical therapy and does not recur. This is so infrequent that it does not justify deferring surgery in the average case.

Diagnosis

Careful history taking is absolutely essential, not only as regards the immediate episode but also related to the whole reproductive history of the bitch. Despite all modern ancillary aids to diagnosis nothing can justify the omission of a thorough clinical examination; quite apart from the question of prognosis it is necessary so far as is possible to assess any intercurrent disease, especially diabetes mellitus, renal disease (as distinct from the effects of pyometra) and cardiac dysfunction.

The average typical case should present little difficulty in diagnosis but additional steps which assist in the less obvious case include:

Radiography

With good technique a reasonably high proportion of cases can be demonstrated by radiography. Problems may arise in two circumstances: the very distended thin-walled uterus which cannot be outlined and is therefore indistinguishable from accumulations of peritoneal fluid due to other causes. In such cases the small intestine is often displaced to the upper and cranial quadrant of the abdomen and this may be regarded as suggestive of a large viscus displacing the gut. The use of air pumped into the peritoneal cavity to improve contrast is contra-indicated because of the high risk of puncturing a pus-filled uterus with, almost invariably, fatal results.

A second, less common, problem is the difficulty of differentiating between a loculated pyometra and a pregnancy as indicated above.

Haematology

In most cases there is a marked neutrophilia with a shift to the left but this must not be regarded as diagnostic per se, since any condition involving infection and/or inflammatory change will produce similar results. It is also recognized that some well-developed cases exist without any increase in the white cell count and that rarely there may be a neutropaenia.

Cytology of uterine fluid

A recent publication (Barrett, 1979) suggests that cytology of intra-uterine fluid, either swabbed from the vagina or withdrawn from the uterus (a dangerous procedure), may be indicative of the degree of toxicity and may be of value in the assessment of prognosis, requirements for after-care, etc. The presence of predominantly normal neutrophils is associated with low-grade toxicity, as in cases of non-toxic mucometra, whereas necrolytic changes in neutrophils, i.e. karyolysis, karyorrhexis and pyknosis, are associated with toxicity.

Serum glucose estimation

It is highly desirable that this should be done routinely to detect cases of incipient diabetes mellitus which would affect both short- and long-term prognosis.

It may be argued that surgery is urgently needed in any case of pyometra but often owners would not consent if aware of possible future problems.

The least serious short-term effect is poor healing and secondary infection of the incision, and if the above investigation has not been carried out this of itself will underline the need for it.

Blood urea or BUN

Similar to serum glucose estimation, this is a highly desirable technique which should be a routine procedure. Values will nearly always be above normal owing to the renal complications in pyometra cases but nonetheless some estimate of kidney function is most useful.

Urinalysis

This is of very limited value. A dilute urine is to be expected owing to the polydipsia and the renal threshold of serum glucose may not have been reached in diabetes cases. Proteinuria is often present owing to contamination of the specimen from vaginal discharges; however catheterization to obtain a clean specimen is contra-indicated, especially in open cases, as there is a risk of introducing infection into the bladder via the catheter.

Cardiac function

This should be assessed mainly clinically. The value of an ECG is likely to be limited. If the exercise tolerance of the patient has been normal prior to the onset of signs of pyometra it is unlikely that cardiac disease of a degree likely to affect the prognosis is present.

Uterine catheterization to obtain a specimen of discharge in closed cases

This is often suggested but in the average case is unlikely to be feasible for two reasons:

1. The anatomy of the vagina and cervix. As will be noted subsequently the vagina of the bitch is surprisingly long, hence precise manipulation of the distal end of a catheter is not easy. The main problem arises from the fact, not yet sufficiently recognized, that the external cervicalos opens in a ventral direction onto the floor of the cranial vagina and so introduction of the catheter into and through the cervical canal is, to say the least, extremely difficult.

2. The nature of the uterine fluid. In the majority of cases the secretion is too thick to pass into and through a catheter of a size which could even remotely possibly be introduced into the uterus.

Renal manifestations of pyometra complex

Many subjects develop degrees of renal disease without experiencing renal failure, although this is always a potential hazard. Failure implies that more than 75% of functional nephrons have been eliminated. In some cases the disease is concomitant and is unrelated in aetiology to pyometra.

Several disease states exist:

Prerenal uraemia

This is the consequence of inadequate perfusion of undamaged glomeruli. In pyometra this may arise due to dehydration or shock following severe vomiting and diarrhoea or depression and reduced fluid intake. This may also occur postsurgically with 'shock' factors like toxaemia, anaesthesia and surgery being responsible, and in particular sequestration of fluid in the operative area.

In the short term this responds to perfusion but in the long term ischaemic tubular disease may develop. Diagnostic features are high serum or plasma urea nitrogen or creatinine in the presence of urine of specific gravity > 1·025 (i.e evidence of continuing nephron function).

Glomerular disease

Detectable swelling of endothelial and mesangial cells, thickening of basement membranes, etc. and various degrees of ischaemic tubular damage are all signs of glomerular disease which is seen to be reversible, in many cases, following ovarohysterectomy. This condition is apparently associated with the deposition of immune complexes.

The degree of proteinuria associated with glomerular disease in pyometra is variable and its measurement is complicated by the contamination of urine with vaginal discharges. In the majority of cases it is thought to be mild. The associated elevation of serum creatinine or BUN may be difficult to differentiate from that associated with prerenal uraemia. A rapid improvement following perfusion would tend to indicate the latter.

Tubular disease

The polydipsia of pyometra is apparently associated with polyuria, the consequence of impaired tubular concentration of urine. The reason for this impairment in the presence of adequate circulatory levels of ADH is unclear. Some equivocal evidence indicates that *E. coli* endotoxin may be responsible, but equally this disability may also be the result of immunological disturbance. There is no evidence to implicate endocrine dysfunction, abnormal potassium or calcium metabolism or obligatory osmotic diuresis associated with the destruction of functional capacity of large numbers of nephrons.

Concomitant renal disease

Whereas renal disease of pyometra aetiology seems generally reversible, pyometra in patients with existent compensated, but irreversible, primary renal failure may precipitate an uraemic crisis.

Differential diagnosis is difficult but the presence of urine with specific gravity < 1·007 tends to indicate a pyometra-related syndrome. Radiography may indicate reduced renal dimensions indicative of non-pyometra aetiology. Gross visible lesions at the time of surgery or biopsy also suggest a non-pyometra cause.

Treatment of pyometra

There can be no doubt at all that the treatment of choice is ovarohysterectomy and, provided it is undertaken at an early stage, it is very well tolerated (*see* 'Prognosis'). However, there will always be a small proportion of cases in which surgery is not feasible, whether due to owner refusal, intercurrent disease or age of the patient, and in some of these medical treatment will be attempted. Numerous treatments have been described over the years with varying success rates.

Medical treatment of pyometra

No single treatment has achieved universal acceptance, the general success rate of medical treatments alone being low. Treatments may be aimed at primary causative factors or at the secondary consequences of disease, or simultaneously at both.

Suggested hormonal treatments aimed at invoking lysis of corpora lutea which are almost invariably present, thereby eliminating at source the progesterone hormone which may have provoked the primary endometrial lesion and maintained the status of myometrial quiescence and flaccidity, are now called into question by the discovery (Coulson, 1979) that the corpus luteum of the bitch is resistant to the lytic effects of single injections of the hormone prostaglandin $F_2\alpha$ so successfully employed in this capacity in other species. However, testosterone given at 25 mg twice weekly may achieve luteolysis secondary to ovarian atrophy, and if this is achieved and cervical relaxation occurs, discharge of contents may be further stimulated by supportive oestrogen therapy and the judicious administration of ecbolics, particularly oxytocin.

Oestrogens may also be used alone to attempt initiation of cervical relaxation and enhanced myometrial contractility but there is a risk that in a proportion of cases their use, and indeed that of any hormone treatment, may be followed by an acutely worsening situation demanding emergency surgical treatment.

In a different context, the administration of oestrogens may result in an apparent improvement of general condition because of the increased resistance of the oestrogen-primed uterus to infection, but in general this aspect of toxicity is tackled by the systemic administration of antibiotics. Elimination thus of secondary bacterial infection may achieve considerable remission of toxic symptoms in both open and closed cases, but antibiotic therapy alone cannot be expected to achieve the resolution of the hormonally caused endometrial disease.

The use of prostaglandins in the treatment of pyometra continues to evoke interest. These drugs are available as synthetic prostaglandin $F_2\alpha$ — dinoprost (Lutalyse — Upjohn) — and the synthetic analogues to dinoprost — cloprostenol (Estrumate, Planate — ICI) and fluprostenol (Equimate — ICI). There is unsubstantiated evidence that cloprostenol may promote cervical relaxation, but it is generally accepted that the major contribution to uterine emptying by these drugs is their stimulation of powerful uterine contraction.

In view of this, and because of the known fragility of the uterine wall in many cases of pyometra, it is suggested that great caution be exercised in the use of prostaglandins in any other than dilated and freely draining cases. A case of uterine rupture following administration of dinoprost at a dose of 0·23 mg/kg was recorded by Jackson (1979).

Published case reports of the usage of prostglandin $F_2\alpha$, particularly dinoprost, have involved too few animals for the formation of clear opinion as to its value. However, there is suggestive evidence that for effect a dose rate of 0·2 to 0·25 mg/kg is required, and in the series reported by Coulson (1981), at a dose rate of 0·25 mg/kg, 15 out of 16 treated bitches responded satisfactorily, of which 5 were subsequently successfully used for breeding.

In cases of failure of hormonal and antibiotic therapy, or as an alternative, a combined surgicomedical approach may be selectively employed, with surgical extirpation of corpora lutea, distension of the cervix or even uterine marsupialization to achieve drainage. Uterine lavage may also be practised in cases of adequate placement of catheters, though this is not easy because of canine cervical configuration.

A technique for the placement of intra-uterine catheters, described by Obel et al. (1981), requires general anaesthesia of the subject in order that the cervix may be visualized through a lighted vaginal speculum and immobilized by the placement of an encircling wire loop. With the aid of fluoroscopy fine plastic catheters are then introduced through the cervix and into each horn, being threaded over removable guide wires. These catheters, which are attached to the vaginal wall with stainless steel sutures, are apparently well maintained, allowing successful drainage for periods of up to 2 weeks. Of the younger bitches so treated, several are reported to have subsequently bred successfully.

Fluid and electrolyte replacement therapy and occasionally the administration of diuretics are indicated in the support of subjects suffering from renal disease either primarily associated with, or simply concomitant with, pyometra. In the case of concomitant renal disease of a compensated but irreversible nature, the occurrence of pyometra itself, or the surgery devolving from it, might precipitate a terminal renal crisis, but in the majority of cases of renal disease which are simply associated with the pyometra syndrome, supportive therapy can be expected to result in full reversal following removal of the toxic source.

In cases of prerenal uraemia in which the ability to concentrate urine is demonstrated by urine of specific gravity $> 1 \cdot 025$, the major requirement is for perfusion of the essentially undamaged glomeruli either by elimination of the 'shock' factors responsible for diverting fluid or, in cases of true dehydration, by fluid replacement. To some extent surgical removal of the toxic source assists by elimination of the aetiology of vomiting, and anorexia, although surgical and anaesthetic procedures may themselves initiate shock reaction in particular by sequestration of fluid in the operative area.

To avoid long-term ischaemic tubular disease in this situation it is advisable at least to ensure the rehydration of dehydrated subjects, with additional treatment consisting of the employment of diuretics to ensure increased renal perfusion, although the claimed benefits of such treatment are difficult to evaluate. Hypertonic dextrose (10-20%) or hypertonic mannitol (20-25%) can be transfused to achieve this effect, or specific diuretics like furosemide or ethacrynic acid can be administered on a daily basis, or even 8-hourly, for several days for as long as adequate hydration and electrolyte replacement therapy is ensured. This can best be achieved by the slow intravenous administration of Hartman's solution B.P. at a rate of 40-50 ml/kg on a daily basis, with appropriate adjustment to meet additional requirements occasioned by persistent vomiting and diarrhoea or reduced thirst in the presurgical phase.

Furosemide and ethacrynic acid, if used, may be administered orally, but preferably intravenously at dose rates recommended by the manufacturers. In the case of furosemide, initial dose rates as high as 8 mg/kg have been reported in use, with treatment repeated 8-hourly according to effect.

The relatively delicate renal changes responsible for pyometra-induced glomerular disease and tubular disease may be difficult to differentiate precisely in the whole animal from changes due to concomitant renal disease of totally separate aetiology. Neither renal shrinkage visible radiographically or during surgery, nor grossly visible renal lesions are indicative of pyometra-induced disease, whereas a urine of specific gravity consistently $< 1 \cdot 007$ tends to indicate the pyometra-induced syndrome of induced diabetes insipidus. Since both glomerular and tubular lesions thus induced, presumably by deposition of immune complexes, are reversed relatively rapidly following removal of the toxic focus, it is unnecessary that the condition be specifically treated medically.

In a few uraemic subjects it is impossible to differentiate simply on the basis of measured blood and urinary parameters between prerenal disease and glomerular nephritis of any aetiology, and in these cases prognosis must be guarded for whatever treatment is offered.

Preoperative medical treatment

It is a very difficult and indeed worrying decision as to whether operation should be deferred to permit some antibacterial therapy. In febrile cases indicative of active bacterial infection a pre-operative course (2 to 3 days) of a suitable antibacterial agent is undoubtedly desirable in open cases; in closed cases the decision is less clear-cut and on balance it would seldom seem wise to defer surgery.

It is sometimes tempting to attempt to improve cardiac function before operating, but the relatively slow response of the canine heart to most drugs in this category probably outweighs its possible value. The continued presence of a toxic focus likewise militates against improved cardiac function.

Prognosis

This should be good in all cases in which operation can be performed at an optimum time. Despite the frequency and routine nature of pyometra surgery, most clinicians would agree that many problems can be met so that these cases are never approached in a complacent frame of mind.

There are a number of factors which will affect the prognosis.

Age of patient

Longevity is largely an inherited characteristic and varies widely from breed to breed. Surgery can usually be recommended if the individual has the possibility of a reasonable survival time post-operatively. Opinions as to the optimum length of this period differ; one year plus has been suggested as an arbitrary figure.

In most breeds surgery can reasonably be recommended up to 11 years of age. After this age great care must be exercised in assessing the general state of health apart from the uterus. The smaller terrier and toy breeds often have a considerable expectation of life — 15 to 17 years is not unusual — thus it may be proper to advise treatment up to 14 years. On the other hand the bull breeds and many of the giant breeds have an average life expectancy of less than 10 years and in these breeds age limits will be set much lower.

Diabetes mellitus detected simultaneously

Whilst many patients survive surgery surprisingly well, delayed wound healing and infection are common. It is seldom feasible to delay operation for a sufficient time to enable a diabetic patient to be balanced on insulin and the appropriate diet prior to surgery, but such therapy must be instigated at the earliest possible stage post-operatively.

Renal disease

If kidney function is impaired, as distinct from the uterine condition, recovery is unlikely. Improvement may occur immediately following hysterectomy but this is seldom maintained and deterioration commences some 7 to 10 days later.

Cardiac disease

Prognosis is similarly affected as for renal dysfunction although a slightly higher proportion of patients do recover and have a reasonable survival time.

ENDOMETRITIS

In dealing with endometritis as a separate entity the authors are aware that this does not conform to Dow's classification (Dow 1957), but clinically there would appear to be justification for this approach.

Endometritis is here defined as a uterus in which pathological change results in a short, thickened organ with a more scanty secretion and no massive fluid accumulation as in pyometra. Two syndromes can be recognized:

Acute endometritis

This occurs in the metoestrous period and in many ways resembles classical pyometra but the presenting signs are quicker and more severe. Affected bitches become acutely ill and owners seldom delay seeking advice longer than 48 hours. Inappetence, thirst, vomiting and profound malaise are usually shown. Vaginal discharge is not copious but is more fluid than the usual pyometra discharge, and is often of a serosanguineous nature and noticeably warm. Abdominal palpation is resented, with muscle guarding.

Response to medical treatment is poor and despite a poor prognosis hysterectomy should be attempted as soon as possible without delaying for the previously recommended investigations. Radiography will not be helpful. On laparatomy a developed peritonitis may already exist. The uterus is usually shorter than even a normal uterus, with very thickened walls and often a rugose appearance. Occasionally the serosa has an almost 'scalded' pitted appearance.

As already indicated, prognosis is poor and no explanation for this syndrome can be offered other than that bacterial permeation and penetration of the uterine wall have occurred at a very early stage.

Chronic endometritis

This presents a totally different picture from the acute form. It usually arises in bitches of early middle life and the signs are relatively mild. General health is often not affected. Because of the insidious course it is not easy to relate the time of onset to the reproductive cycle, but experience suggests that it is probably most often noticed first in late metoestrus. The main, and often only, clinical sign is of a persistent vaginal discharge. This is usually of a mucoid nature and is seldom purulent; the amount varies from day to day. As with any vaginal discharge males are slightly attracted but the bitch is quite unreceptive and sexual advances are seldom vigorous or persistent. As there is often no detectable change in general health owners may delay seeking advice for several weeks.

There is no response to any form of medical treatment and ovarohysterectomy is to be recommended but is rarely urgent. Again, the uterus is short and thickened but with no evidence of active change as in the acute form. Prognosis is very good and despite the apparent absence of systemic signs pre-operatively owners often comment on a marked improvement in health subsequently. Histological changes are typical of a cystic endometrial hyperplasia.

NEOPLASIA

Tumours occur comparatively rarely and are often asymptomatic, their presence being noticed at laparotomy or during routine abdominal palpation; in the latter case precise diagnosis of the organ of origin is often not achieved owing to the absence of related organic signs. Most uterine tumours are benign, leiomyomas probably being the most common type.

THE CERVIX

This is an organ of much importance in the bitch to which comparatively little attention has been paid. The main features of significance to the clinician are:

1. Its inaccessibility per vaginam due to the very long vagina.

2. The direction of the external cervical os. In the non-oestrous and non-parturient bitch the caudal opening of the cervical canal is directed downwards, towards the floor of the cranial vagina. As a consequence of the attachment of the cervix to the roof of the vagina by a midline dorsal fold, it is possible that during oestrus and certainly when dilated at parturition, its direction will become more horizontal in a caudal direction.

Whilst dissection of numerous bitches and careful endoscopic examination of the paracervical area of the anterior vagina of the live subject has confirmed irrefutably the first findings, opportunities for dissecting oestrous and parturient bitches have been few, hence the suggestion of changed direction is largely conjectural. These facts make such procedures as uterine catheterization or intra-uterine deposition of semen not very practicable, if not actually impossible, in the bitch, and even during endoscopic examination identification of the cervix and its os may be complicated by the intrusion of the dorsal median fold and its tubercles into the paracervical area.

The cervix remains relatively closed in normal bitches except during the oestrous cycle and parturition. As mentioned above it opens in some cases of pyometra. It may well be a site from which bleeding occurs during pro-oestrus and in cases of closed pyometra. Careful endoscopic examination of the paracervical region of the anterior vagina has confirmed softening and congestion of mucosal surfaces during the metoestral phase with a patchy hyperaemia apparently associated with rapid exfoliation of epithelium (Lindsay 1978). Failure or delay of relaxation during labour will be referred to later (p. 81).

REFERENCES

Barrett R. P. (1979) Cytology of uterine fluid in a case of pyometra in a dog. *Vet. Med. Small Anim. Clin.* 74, 63.

Coulson A. (1979) Treatment of canine pyometra with dinoprost. *Vet. Rec.* 105, 151.

Coulson A. (1981) Communication to the British Small Animal Veterinary Association Annual Congress, London.

Dow C. (1957) The cystic hyperplasia–pyometra complex in the bitch. *Vet. Rec.* 69, 1409–1415.

Dow C. (1958) *Vet. Rec.* 70, 1102–1110.

Dow C. (1959a) Experimental production of the cystic hyperplasia–pyometra complex in the bitch. *J. Pathol. Bacteriol.* 78, 267–278.

Dow C. (1959b) The cystic hyperplasia–pyometra complex in the bitch. *J. Comp. Pathol.* 69, 237-250.

Jackson P. G. G. (1979) Treatment of canine pyometra with dinoprost. *Vet. Rec.* 105, 131.

Lindsay F. E. F. (1978a) An introduction to endoscopy of the canine bitch post uterine tract. *Pedigree Digest* 5, No. 3, 8–10.

Lindsay F. E. F. (1978b) *Pedigree Digest* 5, No. 4, 8–9.

Obel N., Linde C. and Funkqvist B. (1981) Communication to the British Small Animal Veterinary Association Annual Congress, London.

FURTHER READING

Hardy R. H. and Osborne C. A. (1974) Canine pyometra: pathophysiology, diagnosis and treatment of uterine lesions. *J. Am. Anim. Hosp. Assoc.* 10, 245-267.

Chapter 3

Vagina, Vestibule and Vulva

VAGINA

The vagina of the bitch — here taken to be the total length from the vulva to the cervix, including the vestibule — is very long indeed, e.g. 10–14 cm in a 25-lb bitch. It is thus impossible for the exploring finger to reach the cervix in all except very small bitches and occasionally in medium-sized parturient bitches at the peak of a straining effort (*see Fig. 1*).

There seems to be little doubt that the area of constriction at the demarcation between the vestibule and vagina, the cingulum, which is provided by the constrictor vestibularis muscle, is frequently mistaken for the cervix; as with the cervix itself this muscle is normally contracted except during oestrus and parturition.

Apart from creating problems of diagnosis, e.g. of suspected vaginal tumours and recognizing the stage of labour existing, the very long vagina makes precise vaginal swabbing less easy, and many reputedly vaginal swabs are only vestibular in reality, an important point to remember when investigating the bacterial status of the genital tract. Gentle but prolonged pressure by the swab against the closed constrictor muscle will nearly always result in relaxation which allows the swab to pass cranially some 1–2 in. into the vagina proper from which swabs must be taken if they are to be of any value. Failure of the constrictor vestibularis muscle to relax during oestrus will be discussed later.

The vagina is lined by a relatively tough mucous membrane which shows longitudinal rugae; these are especially apparent during oestrus and parturition. It is possible to recognize digitally the cornified membrane during oestrus and the very marked cyclical changes of mucosal texture can also be recognized with the naked eye at endoscopy, as well as being demonstrated cytologically by smear technique. It would seem that the vagina is relatively resistant to bacterial infection and that this inherent resistance is increased during the oestrous cycle; thus vaginal swabs intended to evaluate the bacterial state of the genital tract should preferably be taken during anoestrus.

The vestibule, in contrast, is lined by smooth mucous membrane; the urethra opens into it just caudal to the caruncle which itself is caudal to the constrictor area. In the light of the history often obtained in evaluating infertile bitches, i.e. that a previous urinary tract infection such as cystitis has existed, the site of the urethral orifice must be regarded as significant in the spread of infection into the vagina. The urethra may also have a role in the persistence of genito-urinary infections.

Anatomical abnormalities of the vagina can be recognized by those experienced in the mating of bitches, despite denials by some veterinary anatomists. Endoscopists have also remarked upon the variability of the direction of the long axis of the vagina, a factor of importance in the avoidance of trauma during insertion of instruments.

The significance of these abnormalities is the difficulty they cause in effective intromission during coitus. The first two described would appear to be related to conformation of the bony pelvis.

1. The so-called 'up and over' vagina is the first of these abnormalities. The vestibule rises at a more acute vertical angle than normal, reaches a peak over the floor of the pelvis then tends to become horizontal or even ventral in direction in extreme cases as it proceeds cranially. The problems caused during attempted intromission are obvious. By digital palpation of very relaxed subjects presenting this variation it is considered that the cause may relate to both angulation of the pelvis and the degree of indentation of the posterior pelvic brim at the point of the pubic symphysis.

2. In a few bitches the vestibule proceeds cranially almost horizontally rather than rising at the normal angle. In these subjects intromission is again impeded as the penis hits the roof of the vagina during thrusting.

3. A state of stenosis at the vestibulovaginal junction has been described (Holt and Sayle, 1981) and implicated as a cause of mating difficulty and vaginitis. This is not a very common condition, and it is uncertain to what extent it may be represented by the failure of relaxation of the constrictor vestibularis muscle.

4. The presence of transverse fibrous bands at the level of the constrictor vestibularis has occasionally been noted in bitches previously examined and known to be free from obstruction. It is assumed that these bands may relate to adhesions consequent upon damage caused by initial examination or following trauma associated with forceps-assisted whelping. The presence of fibrous bands of tissue which are probably remnants of the Müllerian ducts is occasionally found. It is disturbing to note that there is a tendency for this to occur in certain families. The abnormal tissue usually divides the vagina in a vertical plane and is usually situated just cranial to the constrictor area; the extent and thickness of the tissue is very variable. In most cases mating is impossible although successful

mating and whelping has been reported in such a case, also the occurrence of an obstructive dystocia (Herr, 1978) easily corrected by severance of the band. However, although surgical removal of the abnormal tissue can be carried out it is seldom completely successful in permitting breeding. Two cases of virtual bifid vagina are known, resulting from unusually extensive fibrous septa.

Tumours

Vaginal tumours are fairly common and are usually benign. Fibromas, leiomyomas and polyps all occur. Fibromas and leiomyomas are usually located in the vagina proper and are often submucous in site. Clinical signs include vaginal haemorrhage unrelated to the oestrous cycle, bulging of the perineal area or appearance at the vulva. More rarely, unsuspected tumours may become apparent as a cause of obstructive dystocia or may cause episodes of straining, as if in labour or even associated with defaecation. In the latter respect vaginal tumours may cause intrapelvic rectal compression analogous to that caused in the male by prostatic hypertrophy.

Treatment in all cases is surgical and may occasionally require a combined laparotomy or even ovaro-hysterectomy with a vaginal approach. Tumours are often multiple and found the whole length of the vagina from the cingulum to the cervix and their complete removal may require that episiotomy be performed to effect adequate access.

Episiotomy in the bitch is extremely easy. Due to the distance between the anus and vulva a vertical incision is both possible and satisfactory. One blade of a pair of straight scissors can be simply introduced into the vulva and the vestibule and then used to cut through all tissues to the limit of the circumanal tissue. Haemorrhage is surprisingly slight. The operation should never be performed during the oestrous cycle.

In most cases the tumours are well demarcated and encapsulated. The overlying mucosa is incised and the masses shelled out; mucosal incisions are apposed with absorbable sutures. The episiotomy incision is preferably closed in three layers; the mucous membrane and the thick fibro-elastic layers with absorbable material and the skin with monofilament nylon. Healing is usually extremely good.

Polyps

So-called vaginal polyps are quite common in ageing bitches and are nearly always unsuspected until they suddenly appear through the vulva. This situation is usually presented as an emergency, often during the latter part of the oestrous cycle. Depending on the degree of ground contamination the lesion is seen as a small mass of tissue, some 1–2 cm in diameter, occasionally ulcerated, with variable haemorrhage, sometimes masked by dirt from the ground and sometimes seen as a single nodular mass often with a rough surface. Investigation usually demonstrates a long pedicle.

Treatment is surgical and very simple but the technique will be more or less precise according to circumstances. In the very old bitch in which general anaesthesia may be a hazard the technique can be as simple as gently pulling the polyp outwards to expose a length of pedicle, introducing local analgesia into the pedicle, ligating with cat-gut and severing below the ligature. If the bitch is a reasonable anaesthetic risk greater precision can be achieved and greater traction can be applied in the unconscious subject, hence the section can be made fairly high up in the vagina; episiotomy is seldom if ever required. Pedicles are often up to 4 in. in length.

Results are excellent, recurrence is rare and owners are normally most impressed at the speed and simplicity of dealing with what they have regarded as a serious emergency.

Vaginal hyperplasia

This is more usually called vaginal prolapse since vaginal tissue is prolapsed through the vulva. However the term hyperplasia is preferred here since the condition always resolves spontaneously. In some cases it may be more correct to define this as vestibular hyperplasia since the greatest accumulation of oedema is within vestibular and vulval tissues as related to the urethral orifice.

The cause is assumed to be hyperoestrenism which results in massive oedematous hyperplasia of the vaginal mucous lining. Most cases occur during the oestrous cycle, usually in late pro-oestrus, but cases have been seen just prior to parturition, both of these being periods of rising oestrogen levels. There is evidence of breed and even familial incidence. The bull breeds are heavily represented, e.g. bulldogs, bull mastiffs and boxers; Dalmatians have at one time shown a family tendency.

The lesion appears at and through the vulval lips as a glistening mass of vaginal tissue usually covered by smooth epithelium; these masses quickly become traumatized, i.e. dirty and ulcerated, if the owner does not seek prompt advice. The course is invariably one of natural resolution as metoestrus supervenes but with every probability of recurrence at ensuing cycles. Apart from the problem of keeping the tissue clean and undamaged there is little effect on the patient. Both mating and whelping can proceed without problem through the prolapsed mass although whether breeding from such subjects is advisable is another matter.

Treatments have been various. Surgical techniques include resection of the mass and insertion of ring pessaries; the latter being quite futile. Resection is obviously successful during the current cycle but recurrence at the following heat period is quite common. Some veterinarians prefer conservative management of the presenting episode with attention to hygiene and the provision of protective 'pants' until natural remission occurs. This should be followed by consideration of the long-term approach. Ovarohysterectomy will prevent further episodes as will the suppression of further cycles by the use of progestogens.

In the rare cases which arise just prior to whelping there is usually no need for any interference and parturition can proceed normally.

Vaginitis

An infantile vaginitis may be seen in puppies of from 10 weeks to 6 months of age, presenting as a vaginal discharge, usually yellow in colour and with variable evidence of irritation. It is arguable that the condition is truly vaginal since it may sometimes be of solely vestibular siting. Examination of the mucosa only rarely reveals lesions of dog-pox and response to routine systemic antibiotic therapy is usually prompt. Occasionally resistant cases are encountered but these often resolve spontaneously at the onset of first oestrus.

A vaginitis associated with symptoms of irritation and urinary frequency may be encountered in older bitches and was a regular diagnostic feature of cases of vestibulovaginal stricture (Holt and Sayle, 1981). The extent to which vaginitis per se is responsible for the symptomatology of urinary frequency encountered in spayed bitches remains equivocal.

Asymptomatic vaginitis is also encountered in adult bitches under investigation for infertility from which a variety of vaginal bacteria may be isolated.

THE VESTIBULE

This is the site of lesions of two conditions which are recognized regularly.

Dog-pox

This condition has been described fairly fully (Joshua, 1975). Although it is apparently less common in the female (possibly a false impression due to the fact that the lesions are not so readily seen), it nonetheless occurs regularly. Lesions are seen on the vestibular mucosa. They may be found in patients which are apparently asymptomatic in this respect.

When signs do occur they are commonest in the younger age groups, including puppies; signs include vaginal discharge (not invariable) and evidence of irritation such as frequent licking of the vulva or sudden sitting down reminiscent of anal gland problems. Presence of lesions can be confirmed by palpation and/or endoscopy but they are not always easily demonstrated in the conscious animal.

Lesions

Lesions are papular in type, 1 to 1·5 mm in diameter, and may be present as scattered, discrete eruptions or, when numerous and almost contiguous, may appear as a moist, granular mass. Individual lesions often appear haemorrhagic with blood oozing from the ulcerated surface; this is most common with penile lesions. The papules often glisten and give the impression of being vesicular but histologically most are purely aggregations of lymphocytes with no evidence of vesicle formation. A good many cases in bitches appear to resolve spontaneously. There is no specific treatment.

Transmissible venereal tumour (TVT)

Although TVT cannot be described as truly indigenous it does occur, if infrequently, in Great Britain. It is seen in areas around seaports, due to the illegal landing of dogs, and in dogs soon after they leave quarantine as the period between infection and the development of obvious lesions can be many months. Transmission is truly venereal.

In bitches the lesion develops on the vestibular mucosa and tends to progress in an annular fashion. The lesion is proliferative and the surface is roughened and bleeds easily. The commonest sign is of a haemorrhagic vaginal discharge and consequent licking by the bitch. A history of mating several months previously is suggestive, especially if to a roaming male. Signs can develop at any stage of the cycle.

Diagnosis is by palpation and endoscopy, possibly exploratory surgery, and should be reinforced by histological examination which is pathognomonic. Surgical treatment can be attempted and comprises resection of the affected area of mucosa; surprisingly drastic resections can be performed with a reasonable prospect of success. Metastasis is not common but has been recorded.

VULVA

The vulva of the puppy is a small organ decorated by a tuft of hair until puberty approaches. It should start to enlarge during the prepubertal period (usually 4 to 8 months) and following tumefaction during the first oestrous period should assume an adult form. In some bitches the vulva remains infantile in size and type in adult life and may remain so or later become recessed into surrounding tissue. Spaying prior to the first heat period prevents full anatomical development of the vulva.

Atretic vulvas, whatever the cause, are liable to cause problems. Urine scalding of the surrounding skin results in a perivulval dermatitis, ulceration and secondary bacterial infection. The clinical signs are often severe out of all proportion to the lesion. Many bitches show extreme discomfort with continuous licking, sudden turning round and sitting down and even occasional yelping or whimpering. Affected tissues are exceptionally sensitive on handling.

The lesions are very resistant to the customary forms of treatment since it is impossible to remove the cause, i.e. the contact and friction of tissues. Oestrogen therapy to induce tumefaction of vulval lips produces only a transient improvement. In some cases a longer-term and more considerable improvement can be affected by the employment of imaginative techniques of plastic surgery, but in others the vulval tissue may be so deeply inset between the thighs that little improvement can be achieved. Wherever possible, surgery should aim to simultaneously achieve resection of inflamed perivulvar tissues and eversion of vulval lips, although to effect the latter it is sometimes necessary to enlarge the vulval opening by performing a partial episiotomy and suturing mucosa to skin edges.

The condition is peculiarly distressing in that the lesions, though not in themselves life-threatening, may result in requests for euthanasia of otherwise healthy subjects. Although a proportion of cases occur in entire bitches, the spaying of prepubertal bitches is responsible in many instances. Avoidance of this condition is implicit in the advocacy of postpubertal spaying.

Vulval hyperplasia

The vulva and perivulvar tissues are unusually prominent in some breeds, e.g. boxer, but this should not give cause for concern. Excessive tumefaction of the vulva and vestibule may coincide with oestrus and the immediate prepartum period and need not present a barrier to either mating or whelping. The condition is assumed to be a manifestation of oestrogen sensitivity.

REFERENCES

Herr S. (1978) Persistent post-cervical band as a cause of dystocia in a bitch. *Vet. Med. Small Anim. Clin.* **73**, 1533.
Holt P. E. and Sayle B. (1981) Congenital vestibulo-vaginal stenosis in the bitch. *J. Small Anim. Pract.* **22**, 67–75.
Joshua J. O. (1975) 'Dog-pox' – some clinical aspects of an eruptive condition of certain mucous surfaces in dogs. *Vet. Rec.* **96**, 300–302.

Chapter 4

Oestrous Cycle

The bitch is unique among domestic pets in being monoestrous, i.e. there is only one oestrous cycle in a complete breeding cycle which lasts, on average, for 6 months. The duration of this, however, is subject to considerable variation. Four phases are recognized:

1. *Anoestrus,* a period of sexual quiescence. Duration in an average cycle is about 15 weeks.

2. *Pro-oestrus,* the period of vaginal bleeding. The bitch is rarely sexually receptive although experienced mature brood bitches will occasionally accept service. Duration is exceedingly variable, averaging 8 to 13 days.

3. *Oestrus.* This is the phase of acceptance; vaginal discharge becomes less bloody and even colourless. Duration is variable, averaging 4 to 7 days.

The second and third phases comprise the so-called 'season' or 'heat', or the bitch may be said to be 'in use'.

4. *Metoestrus.* Assuming ovulation has occurred the bitch will be under luteal influence for a period of 6 to 10 weeks. Corpora lutea should regress at about 42 days but may persist for longer.

PHYSIOLOGY OF THE OESTROUS CYCLE

Among the domesticated species the cyclic sexual patterns of the canine female are distinctively different. Even in comparison with wild canine species, the domesticated bitch, despite obvious similarities, remains distinctive, exhibiting usually two rather than one 'season' per annum and having no noticeable link with climatic factors.

Some confusion has arisen and remains about application to the bitch of terminology more appropriate to other species, but there is now general agreement that the bitch be classified as seasonally monocyclic or seasonally monoestrous; this descriptive terminology relates to the fact that in the bitch each episode of sexual activity is separated by a prolonged anoestrous period of apparent sexual quiescence. Although protracted periods of sexual quiescence are not unique to the bitch, in all other domesticated species exhibiting a seasonal habit each 'season' of sexual activity comprises, in the absence of supervening pregnancy, several cycles of ovarian changes. This is not the case in the bitch which exhibits only a single cycle of ovarian changes during each 'season' of sexual activity. Also, in contrast to polyoestrous species, each phase of this cycle of ovarian and hormonal change is manifest by distinctively protracted external symptoms.

Notwithstanding these dissimilarities, the basic mechanisms of control of ovarian activity in the bitch are assumed to be similar to those operating in other species, although precise factors influencing the awakening of ovarian activity after prolonged quiescence, or indeed the factors responsible for the imposition of so protracted a quiescence remain to be elucidated. In respect of this latter feature, it should be stated that one school of thought, in presenting an accumulation of evidence based on hormonal assay and vaginal and uterine cytology, discounts the prolonged anoestrus as a time of true quiescence, seeing it rather as a period of continuous, if low-grade, ovarian and uterine activity developing progressively towards the next cycle of ovarian awakening (Jochle and Anderson, 1977). Because basic measurements of hormonal parameters have not been continued beyond the phases of obvious high-level ovarian activity it remains difficult to substantiate these claims, but with the application of more refined techniques of hormonal assay there is continuous reassessment of these features.

For practical purposes the bitch ovary may be assumed, as in other species, to be controlled by the pituitary release of gonadotrophins. The inter-relationship of various controlling factors upon such release is now known to be far more complex than was formerly hypothesized, and the full extent of hypothalamic sensitivity to circulating blood levels of steroid hormones alone remains to be elucidated. However, it is already apparent that the negative feedback effects of ovarian and possibly adrenal steroid hormones are both subtle and precise (Lamming et al., 1979), placing in question the rationality of many popular hormonal medical treatments.

In the crudest of terms the pituitary release of follicle-stimulating hormone (FSH) may still be considered responsible for the initiation of high-level ovarian activity at the commencement of each cycle, with maturation of Graafian follicles and secretion by them of oestrogens. However, carefully constructed hormone profiles have revealed ascending blood levels of plasma oestrogens commencing during late anoestrus and preceding the onset of pro-oestrous symptoms. This suggests an initial growth of follicles pre-dating the FSH release, traditionally associated with ovarian follicular development and the production of oestrogens.

The outward appearance of symptoms during pro-oestrus, that is, the period classified as preceding sexual receptivity, is one of the most distinctive features of the canine oestrous cycle. During this phase of ovarian follicular growth and oestrogen production, considerable tissue growth occurs throughout the genital tract, being most marked externally by reddening, swelling and turgidity of vulval lips and the appearance of the sanguineous vaginal discharge. The appearance of this vaginal bleeding, eventually established to be due to the loss of red cells by diapedesis into the uterine lumen, was initially the cause of considerable misunderstanding of bitch reproductive physiology, being equated by analogy with primates with a phase of uterine mucosal destruction rather than development. This misconception is still occasionally encountered when, in lay terminology, pro-oestrus is described as 'breaking down' rather than 'in heat', which more accurately reflects the warm touch of the turgid vulva.

Plasma oestrogen levels have been recorded rising to a peak in late pro-oestrus (*Fig.* 2), thereafter declining, the attainment of this peak just preceding a considerable measurable 'surge' increase in plasma levels of the second gonadotrophin, luteinizing hormone (LH) (*Fig.* 2) released from the pituitary to stimulate the rupture of mature Graafian follicles in the ovary. Peak levels of this gonadotrophin are measurable for a variable

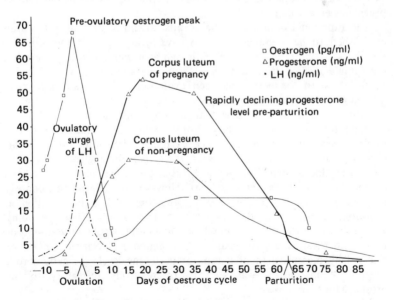

Fig. 2. Plasma hormone profiles of the bitch from several sources and based on a classic 63-day gestation.

period overlapping the final 2 days of pro-oestrus and the first 4 days of standing oestrus which presumably accounts for the clinical observation of somewhat protracted ovulation in some bitches.

Coincident with this period of transition from visible pro-oestrus to standing oestrus when vulval swelling diminishes and sanguineous discharge ceases or is reduced, there is also a measureable increase in plasma progesterone levels, even preceding ovulation and the formation of a fully secretory corpus luteum. This initial low level is assumed to be of follicular origin, but following formation of corpora lutea, plasma progesterone levels rise dramatically attaining peaks sometimes as early as the 7th day of oestrus, but usually by the 25th to 30th day irrespective of pregnancy, the levels measured during pregnancy being, however, statistically higher. Thereafter there is gradual decline of measured plasma levels although corpora lutea retain the appearance of activity. It is apparent from recent experimental work that this continuing activity is attributable to luteotropic support from the pituitary, being interrupted by hypophysectomy unless substituted by the immediate supply of exogenous LH.

In the non-bred bitch this post-ovulatory phase of continuing luteal function – metoestrus – is of variable duration, variously quoted as lasting between 30 and 84 days. Recent work assessing continuing luteal function on the basis of retention of plasma progesterone levels above 1 ng/ml suggests the duration to be habitually of the order of 84 days, in contrast to the much shorter 65-day period of the corpus luteum of pregnancy (*Fig. 2*).

The functional duration of the corpus luteum of pregnancy has been established to be a minimum of 56 days, ovariectomy before this day invariably precipitating abortion, although as in non-pregnancy there is a measurable decline from peak levels from approximately the 30th day post-oestrus. In the period between ovulation and attainment of peak plasma progesterone levels a measured surge coincident with implantation is considered indicative of a placental gonadotrophic factor.

Prepartum a further relatively abrupt decline in plasma progesterone levels is suggestive of the existence of unidentified luteolysins. In this context, the role of known luteolysins like prostaglandins remains enigmatic. Experimentally, the luteolysin prostaglandin $F_2\alpha$ has been demonstrated to be an abortifacient. However its role in this context remains contentious since the injudicious use of $F_2\alpha$ has resulted in symptoms of nausea and distress. Controlled use over a 72-hour period by intramuscular injection has procured apparently satisfactory luteolysis in late metoestrus and pregnancy (Concannon and Hansel, 1977). As assessed by measurement of plasma progesterone levels the early corpus luteum of metoestrus was seen to be relatively refractory to the prostagladin $F_2\alpha$.

In the untreated prepartum bitch the phase of decline of plasma progesterone levels coincides with a measurable upsurge in plasma oestrogen levels and, in the immediate prepartum period, with a measurable increase in plasma corticoid level suggesting that, as in other species, there may exist in the bitch a mechanism for labour induction involving maternal and/or fetal adrenals.

Of most practical clinical significance in the bitch, relative to other species, is the protracted functional life span of the corpus luteum of non-pregnancy. To this has been attributed both peculiarities of bitch uterine pathology and several well-defined clinical behaviour syndromes. In respect of the latter, however, there is increasing evidence that yet more complex hormone interactions exist, and the role in this context of the pituitary hormone prolactin remains to be elucidated.

Measurement of plasma prolactin levels in the prepartum phase reveals a negative correlation with declining progesterone levels, and elevated levels of prolactin are also seen to persist throughout the period of lactation, which can be prolonged artificially by systemic administration of the hormone. Prolactin is not considered to be luteolytic but it is assumed to be responsible for the support of lactation. Furthermore it is hypothesized that lactation in the late metoestrous bitch may be the result of pituitary secretion of prolactin in response to the stimulus of declining plasma progesterone levels.

CLINICAL AND PRACTICAL ASPECTS OF OESTROUS CYCLIC HABIT

Anoestrus

Bitches should be physically and behaviourally normal at this stage. The duration of anoestrus is, like the other phases, subject to considerable variation, from as little as 7 weeks to one year or more. In some breeds it is recognized as being longer than average.

Breeders have long maintained that bitches which habitually come on heat at intervals of 4 months or less are likely to be non-breeders but, unlike most other old wives' tales, this could have a logical basis. If a bitch fails to ovulate there will be no corpora lutea, hence no luteal phase, so reducing an average cycle by 6 to 8 weeks.

Whilst many dermatologists deny that there is any correlation between the reproductive cycle and coat change, most breeders of long-coated varieties would disagree. Moult usually starts in mid- to late anoestrus and the new coat grows in, often surprisingly rapidly, so that the bitch is in full coat during or shortly after her oestrous cycle. Experienced breeders can predict the approximate date of onset of pro-oestrus by the stage of coat growth.

Pro-oestrus

Bitches may show some behavioural change for about 2 weeks prior to the onset of vaginal bleeding; this consists mainly in a change in urination pattern with greatly increased frequency of urination, often with evidence of territory marking. Coincidentally males show a marked increase in interest, mainly of an investigatory nature and with only very tentative attempts to mount which will be vigorously rebuffed. Experienced stud dogs and dogs living with the bitch lose interest when bleeding commences but become attentive again in late pro-oestrus.

Pro-oestrus is classically the stage of vaginal bleeding but examination of smears prepared for cytological estimation of cyclical phases confirms the presence of red blood corpuscles in vaginal discharge for some days before and after bleeding is readily apparent. It is important to realize that the continued presence of even visible blood staining is entirely compatible with the progress of oestrus as judged by other cytological elements.

It must also again be emphasized that endometrial changes during pro-oestrus are in no way analogous to primate menstruation and the source of bleeding is entirely different. Confusion on this matter remained until as recently as 1931 when it was established, by Evans and Cole, that the bleeding is the result of loss of erythrocytes into the uterine lumen by diapedesis. It seems likely that cervical and cranial vaginal mucosal tissues, which have been reported by endoscopists (Lindsay, 1978) to be swollen and oedematous at this stage, may also be sites of erythrocyte loss.

The onset of vulval swelling is variable; it sometimes precedes bleeding by several days, sometimes coincides with it and is sometimes delayed until oestrus is impending.

The duration of pro-oestrus is extremely variable, hence the frequent failure of rule-of-thumb methods of estimating the time for mating. Duration varies from 0–28 days with an average of 8–13 days. Many figures have been quoted for the duration of the phases of the oestrous cycle but these are usually related to a particular colony being studied in which breed and management are uniform and there is often some genetic similarity. Likewise in kennels which practise line and/or in-breeding there is a good deal of uniformity in the pattern of the cycle, hence the success and breeding management based on long knowledge of the strain concerned, e.g. 'I always mate them on the 11th day'. Even in these circumstances variations can arise not only between individuals but from season to season in the one individual. A good example is that of a bitch usually successfully mated between her 12th and 15th days but which, on a subsequent occasion, was not ready until her 29th day when she was mated and conceived. At the following heat this bitch mated herself to a mongrel on her 7th day!

The figure of nil for the duration of pro-oestrus requires some elabora-tion, relating to the cycles which are described as silent or colourless heats. It has been suggested that the explanation is that a mild pro-oestrus has been missed and that it must always occur. However, this is an unsatisfactory explanation, since many experienced breeders anxiously waiting for a particular bitch to come on heat examine them daily with some care and are most unlikely to miss even faint signs. The pattern in such cases is for the bitch to show vulvovaginal swelling, the vulva appearing moist and active; the discharge, which is scanty, is of a colourless mucoid nature or at most faintly pink-tinged. Experienced males in contact show immediate interest and the bitch is receptive from 1 to 4 days after the first signs are noted. Breeders frequently wait for colour to appear only to find that the brief cycle has terminated in 5–8 days. The correct advice in these cases is to try the bitch daily from the first day on which signs are noticed and to mate her at 48-hour intervals for as long as she will accept service; such matings are usually fertile. Some bitches never show pro-oestral bleeding but some interpose a silent heat between otherwise normal cycles.

The degree of pro-oestral bleeding varies. In some breeds a heavy blood loss is frequent, e.g. in German shepherd dogs, Salukis and St. Bernards. Occasionally the loss is sufficient to produce anaemia and if this recurs at every cycle it is an indication for ovarohysterectomy.

Undoubtedly there is a degree of genetic control in oestrous cycle patterns which can be of assistance in advising on apparent departures from normal. (*See* Chapter 5.)

Oestrus

Although the average duration of oestrus is 4–7 days, bitches are clearly recognized which can be mated on only one day of the cycle whether due to the female acceptance phase or male interest. Most bitches are mateable for 4 or 5 days and in some oestrus persists for 9 or even 10 days.

Oestrus is traditionally described as the phase of acceptance but this criterion is by no means always reliable. Not only is libido very variable between both breeds and individuals, but the fact that, in controlled breeding programmes, natural selection is abolished is a vitally important factor in assessing acceptance behaviour. Many bitches will vigorously reject, or at least passively resist, the attentions of one male but show an enthusiastic acceptance response to another.

Recognition of oestrus depends upon several criteria: vulval discharge becomes less haemorrhagic, even colourless, though variations occur and some bitches show colour until they pass into metoestrus. Vulvovaginal swelling is maximal and soft, the best site for assessing this being the perineal vagina. Behavioural changes occur, with special reference to the tail-turning reflex. Even bitches of poor libido usually respond with some tail movement to gentle massage of the perineum, and keen bitches may adopt an exaggerated standing posture with very marked deflection of the tail.

Vaginal cytology

It is well recognized that changes in vaginal cytology can be helpful in estimating the stage of the cycle; this is of value to inexperienced owners and is a simple technique which can be easily carried out in the daily routine of practice. (Schutte, 1967.) Relative to the sophistication of diagnostic techniques based on vaginal cytological examinations in the human, little use has been made of cellular monitoring in the bitch other than to follow cyclical phases and particularly to pinpoint the time of ovulation. In some laboratories sufficient data have been accumulated to permit the application to the bitch of diagnostic indices comparable to those used in the human field, but no widespread clinical advantage has yet accrued from this (Schutte 1967, Dore, 1978).

It has been suggested that, for purposes of realistic evaluation of vaginal cytological patterns, deep vaginal sampling is necessary. However, comparative examination of anterior vaginal and vestibular vaginal material from the bitch demonstrates this not to be the case, although reports of vaginal endoscopic examination confirm anterior vaginal mucosal changes to be more grossly remarkable.

Regardless of the site of swabbing, however, it is noteworthy that for diagnostic purposes the advantages of serial sampling over single-sample examination are universally accepted. Sampling techniques described include gentle scraping of vestibular mucosa with glass microslides, wooden spatulae, glassrods or small curettes (e.g. the curette end of a groove director); the removal of anterior vaginal fluids by glass pipette; the instillation of saline to provide vaginal washings; and the use of saline-moistened swabs. In all cases the necessity for gentle handling of material is emphasized, both to avoid trauma to the subject and to minimize misleading distortion of the cytological picture. It seems probable that in experienced hands any of these collection techniques can be utilized satisfactorily.

Smears prepared in routine fashion from the available material are either fixed in alcohol/ether for immediate staining and examination, or else fixed in polyethylene glycol/spirit/acetic acid if they are to be stored or transported before staining.

Staining with modified Schorr's trichrome method probably produces the clearest differentiation between keratinized and non-keratinized cells, but for routine examination of serial samples on a practice basis simpler techniques may be used. In most circumstances Leishman's staining technique is adequate. The keeping quality of the slides is obviously affected by the degree of care taken over the final stages of drying and mounting.

Method (Leishman's)

1. Fix in absolute alcohol and ether (equal parts) for 30 minutes.

2. Stain with undiluted Leishman's solution for 1 minute.
3. Dilute with equal volume of distilled water and leave for 10-15 minutes.
4. Wash and differentiate in distilled water.
5. Dry and mount.

Microscopical appearance of smears

Pro-oestrus

The proportions of several cell types varies with the phase of pro-oestrus, in particular the numbers of red blood corpuscles which may in very early and very late pro-oestrus be relatively few. In the early stages nucleated epithelial cells predominate, giving way in the later stages to more cornified cells with pyknotic nuclei. Leucocytes visible in early pro-oestrus become progressively fewer in number as the phase moves towards oestrus.

Oestrus

Smears are initially not dissimilar to those of late pro-oestrus. Generally there is marked absence of leucocytes and red blood cells, though occasionally the latter persist throughout. The predominant cell type is the anuclear, keratinized epithelial cell; towards late oestrus these cells present a wrinkled, ragged-edged appearance as they degenerate.

Metoestrus

An abrupt change in cell type is found as numerous polymorphonuclear leucocytes appear, predominating in early metoestrus. There is re-appearance of nucleated epithelial cells and virtually total absence of red blood cells, except in cases of prolonged bleeding.

Anoestrus

Merging with the late metoestrus phase there is a diminution of polymorphonuclear leucocytes, although some may be present. A predominance of large, nucleated epithelial cells with relatively few non-nucleated cells is to be found.

Interpretation

The subject is reviewed by Dore (1978). Although all bitches follow the same basic pattern there are some variations as noted, and individuals are observed to exhibit their own particular patterns in successive cycles. Because of this degree of individual variation it is impossible to impose absolute diagnostic values, but in general it is considered that for the majority of bitches ovulation coincides with the phase of oestrous cycle at which the ratio of keratinized to non-keratinized epithelial cells equals or exceeds 3 : 2. Individual cases may be noted to ovulate without achieving this ratio and only knowledge gained by sampling serially during several cycles can be utilized in these cases. In others the ratio may be seen to increase beyond the supposed optimum day, in which case repeat mating should be performed. To obtain greatest advantage from serial sampling, it is advisable that frequency be increased from every third day during early pro-oestrus to daily during the critical oestrous phase.

In cases of persistent failure to conceive and in which late ovulation is assumed likely, the retrospective system of assessment of Holst and Phemister (1975) may be useful for assessing the likely peak of oestrus in the next cycle, assuming the bitch to behave regularly. In their series of 31 bitches, ovulation as indicated by a measured upsurge in plasma levels of LH was seen to occur regularly 8 (SE 0·03) days before termination of the oestrous period as determined cytologically, the end-point being the day on which a marked decrease in the proportion of keratinized superficial epithelial cells was observed. This relationship of ovulation to end-point was seen to be fixed regardless of the duration of pre-ovulatory oestrus as judged cytologically, although in the majority of cases that period was of approximately 4 days' duration.

Hormonal control of oestrus

Induction of oestrus

Since the use for breeding of bitches of anything other than regular cyclic habits is ethically questionable, the application of techniques for oestrus induction is limited. Administration of oestrogens by mouth or parenterally invariably provokes changes within the female reproductive tract and psyche, but the degree of effect is dose-dependent and variable.

Vaginal cytological examination may confirm these changes with the appearance of typically pro-oestrous smears, but these are not accompanied by ovarian follicular development so that the administration of oestrogens alone cannot reliably be assumed to be capable of inducing anything other than symptomatic oestrus. There remains a degree of reservation in the expression of this opinion as claims are frequently made for the total efficacy of this simple technique, but it seems particularly improbable that anything so uncontrolled as a single depot injection of oestrogens could be usefully employed thus, since the use of these drugs in the context of treatment of misalliance in the bitch (at dose rates of 5–10 mg oestradiol benzoate or 10–20 mg stilboestrol diproprionate) sometimes provokes symptoms of overt oestrus with prominent vulval swelling for periods as long as 6–8 weeks.

Induction of ovulatory oestrus

This can be achieved by the use of follicle stimulating hormone (FSH) alone or in combination with luteinizing hormone (LH). Wright (1980), in a review of the various regimes recorded, reports the tremendous variability of response and in particular the relative refractoriness of prepubertal subjects. His suggestion for greatest success is dose adjustment on an individual basis as assessed by vulval and vaginal changes and rising serum oestrogen measurements, although the latter is not practicable at general practice level. A simple regime is the daily administration over a 3 week period of up to 200 i.u. of FSH followed by up to 300 i.u. of LH on the day of service. A shorter course with a claimed 80% success rate advocates subcutaneous or intramuscular injection of FSH daily for 9 days at 44 i.u./kg followed by 500 i.u. LH on the 10th day, or on the first day of observable oestrus, this usually being within 2 weeks of commencement of treatment.

Induction of ovulation

Induction of ovulation without signs of overt oestrus can be achieved by administration at intervals of 48 hours of two injections of up to 500 i.u. of LH, a technique which could conceivably be utilized in conjunction with the controlled administration of oestrogens.

Under field conditions, none of these techniques offers the degree of success which may be achieved in the controlled experimental environment.

Postponement or suppression of oestrus

This can be achieved by the administration of male hormones or progestogens, and the use of the latter in particular is now widely practised. Their effect is achieved by an ill-defined suppression of pituitary secretion of gonadotrophins, and reservation about their use relates both to the wide range of side-effects attributable to their progestogenic component and to their formulation in some cases for use as slow-release depot injections. It must, however, be stated that this use of male hormones and progestogens has been extensively practised in greyhound racing establishments where, under well-controlled conditions, the advantages of maintenance of racing form by avoidance of pro-oestrus and oestrus have been found to outweigh the risks of induced pathology in a small proportion of cases.

The concept of *postponement of oestrus* rather than its suppression relies upon prejudgement of the time of onset of pro-oestrus, allowing for the commencement of therapy before the onset of signs. Dosage recommendations for drugs in common use are shown in Table 1. Used thus, these drugs prevent the onset of pro-oestrus and the animal may be assumed likely to resume cyclic activity after its normal anoestrus interval.

Table 1. Drugs and dose recommendations for the postponement of oestrus

Medroxyprogesterone acetate (subcutaneous injection)
(28 mg/ml)
Administered 6–8 weeks before oestrus.
  Up to 25 kg body weight – 2 x 28 mg.
  Up to 50 kg body weight – 2–4 x 28 mg.

Medroxyprogesterone acetate (oral)
(5 mg tabs)
Administered in anoestrus at least 5 days before pro-oestrus.
  Up to 25 kg body weight – 5 mg daily for as long as required.
  Over 25 kg body weight – 10 mg daily for as long as required.

Megestrol acetate (oral)
(5 mg and 20 mg tabs)
Administered 7–14 days before anticipated pro-oestrus.
  0·5 mg/kg daily for up to 40 days *or*
  initial 40-day course as above followed by
  0·1 to 0·2 mg/kg twice weekly for 4 months.

Proligestone (subcutaneous injection)
(100 mg/ml)
Administered in anoestrus not more than one month before oestrus.
  Up to 33 mg/kg to a maximum of 600 mg.

By the repeated application of this method at appropriate intervals, usually on a 6-monthly basis, total avoidance of cyclic activity may be achieved, but not without subsequent risk of failure of cyclic normality following the eventual cessation of therapy.

The alternative system of control is by *suppression* of the overt symptoms of pro-oestrus by the administration of similar progestogens or male hormones at dose levels higher than those utilized in the postponement technique (Table 2). This implies in many cases the creation of high blood levels of progestogens in uterine tissues already primed with oestrogens and so may be assumed to carry an increased risk of induced uterine pathology.

Drug preparations in common use

Apart from testosterone which may be administered orally or by injection but which has been largely superceded, the drugs available for use by either technique are progesterone, its derivatives and synthetic substitutes, many of which are also available for use orally or in parenteral formulations designed for slow-release depot utilization.

Against the convenience of single-dose administration of depot compounds must be offset the inevitable risks associated with the presence in

*Table 2. **Drugs and dose recommendations for the suppression of oestrus***

Medroxyprogesterone acetate (oral)
(5 mg tabs)
Administered at commencement of pro-oestral bleeding.
  Up to 25 kg body weight — 10 mg daily for 4 days then 5 mg daily for 12 days.
  Over 25 kg body weight — double above dose.

Megestrol acetate (oral)
(5 mg and 20 mg tabs)
Administered at onset of pro-oestrus.
  2 mg/kg for 8 days *or*
  2 mg/kg for 4 days followed by 0·5 mg/kg for 16 days.

Proligestone (subcutaneous injection)
(100 mg/ml)
Administered at any phase of pro-oestrus/oestrus, but preferably in early pro-oestrus.
  Up to 33 mg/kg body weight to a maximum of 600 mg.

the body of irretrievable, slowly metabolized hormones having both variable duration and a range of side-effects. It is this use of progesterone and medroxyprogesterone compounds which has been associated with the most frequently recorded cases of induced uterine pathology, prolonged anoestrus, increased body weight, altered weight distribution and temperamental and behavioural changes including false pregnancy and lactation. Most of these effects are usually associated with the metoestrus phase of normal cyclic activity and the more recently introduced synthetic agents are claimed to be relatively free of these specifically progestogenic effects, while retaining their antigonadotrophic activity. Such claims, with only a low risk of undesirable effects on the endometrium and ovaries and only medium duration action so that cumulation is unlikely even after multiple dosage, together with its suitability for use at any stage of the oestrous cycle, are made for the new injectable proligestone and for the progestin delmadinone acetate which may be administered by injection or orally. Delmadinone, however, although occasionally usefully employed in the treatment of pseudocyesis and behavioural symptoms of metoestrus, is associated less with oestrus control than with control of male hypersexuality, its powerful anti-androgen activity being attributed to effects exerted on the hypothalamus and pituitary.

More rapidly metabolized progestogens formulated for oral administration, though more laborious to use on a daily basis, permit the exercise of a greater degree of control, thus avoiding the risks associated with the use of depot injections. The best-known progestogen in this category is megestrol acetate which can be used on short- or long-term bases and at relatively high or low weight-related dose levels to achieve the degrees of oestrus control previously referred to as *suppression* and *postponement*.

Although apparently safe in use at recommended dose levels this drug is not specifically antigonadotrophic, rather having a wide range of progestogenic side-effects, some of which have resulted in its useful application in the treatment of false pregnancy and lactation, in the treatment of oestrogen-dependent mammary tumours and in the treatment of some cases of misalliance in bitches already undergoing medication with the drug.

In male dogs megestrol acetate has been successfully employed in the treatment of a proportion of cases exhibiting symptoms of hypersexuality and aggression, a combination of antigonadotrophic and progestogenic effects being assumed responsible for its effectiveness.

Less satisfactory side-effects include increased appetite and weight gain, especially in cases of prolonged dosage, and in the bitch the association of megestrol acetate therapy with uterine changes, including pyometra, has been reported. The weight of evidence for the bitch, however, points to therapeutic dose levels being well below those required experimentally to induce cystic endometrial hyperplasia, mucometra or pyometra. The results of clinical surveys even suggest a higher natural incidence of pyometra found in bitches routinely presented for spaying than in bitches previously medicated with megestrol acetate at various therapeutic dose levels.

Experimental evidence points to the overall safety of megestrol acetate when used within therapeutic limits, to its lack of teratogenic or pregnancy prolonging effects if administered inadvertently at time of conception, and also to its total lack of effect on subsequent fertility and breeding performance. These claims are similar to those already quoted for the injectable progestogen proligestone which, as the most recent addition to the market, appears to rival megestrol acetate most closely in terms of efficacy in the sphere of oestrus control in the bitch.

FALSE PREGNANCY

As has been mentioned earlier, the reproductive cycle of the bitch is unique amongst those of domestic pets in that it is monoestrous. The genital organs go through a complete breeding cycle, whether the bitch is mated or not, with all the associated hormonal changes. Since the bitch is a spontaneous ovulator, corpora lutea develop in the ruptured Graafian follicles with the consequence that there is a progestational phase of variable duration when the animal is under luteal influence, i.e. metoestrus. There is no di-oestrus phase in the bitch, anoestrus succeeding metoestrus and having a duration of some 15 weeks in an average cycle.

In some bitches little, if any, observable evidence of metoestrus occurs but a very high proportion do show recognizable signs which are to a variable degree abnormal and even pathological. These signs are at the least an inconvenience and at the worst a source of considerable worry to owners and are apparently distressing to the bitch. It is a problem on which veterinary advice is frequently sought. Although the condition is self-limiting as the cycle passes into quiescence, its duration is very variable and treatment meets with differing success.

Recorded surveys of false pregnancy in the bitch are largely based on cases presented to clinicians for attention. Almost certainly the incidence is far higher than most published figures suggest as many bitch owners, especially dog breeders/exhibitors, are quite familiar with the phenomenon and do not seek veterinary advice unless the signs are extreme.

Although false pregnancy is usually regarded as a single clinical entity, several different manifestations can be recognized and treatment must be adjusted to the type involved.

Gross symptoms suggestive of pregnancy

Soon after oestrus ends the bitch shows several changes which include some or all of the following: increased appetite; changes in temperament and behaviour which include sluggishness, loss of interest in exercise and increase in demonstration of affection. There is often increase in body weight which may be either generalized, limited to abdominal distension, or both. Abdominal distension becomes obvious at an earlier stage than is possible in true pregnancy, and if the bitch has been mated the owner is convinced she is in whelp despite advice to the contrary. These signs occur after every oestrous cycle but often vary considerably in intensity. Although some hypertrophy of mammary tissue may occur it is seldom marked and rarely ends in lactation in this syndrome.

Treatment

Treatment of this form is often unsatisfactory and is usually by use of hormones. Androgens are generally of little value although there are reports of the successful use of delmadinone.

Although no statistics can be presented to support the hypothesis, clinical observation suggests that it is this type of false pregnancy patient which has a predisposition to pyometra. Some workers deny that there is any connection between the existence of pathological metoestrous phases and subsequent uterine disease, but published work has not included a classification of the varying manifestations of false pregnancy such as is attempted here.

In most cases of this type of false pregnancy the abdominal distension disappears uncannily suddenly at about the 49th day post-oestrus. This accounts for the frequent history given to the practitioner that 'The bitch was obviously in whelp but we came down this morning and she must have aborted and eaten the puppies'. Although uterine changes have been described for metoestrus the degree is insufficient to account for the obvious abdominal enlargement and explanations for the very sudden decrease have not been given. Clearly it is associated with the regression of luteal tissues in the 42- to 49-day period but this seems insufficient to account for this phenomenon.

Vaginal discharge at this stage is uncommon but does occasionally occur; it is usually of scanty quantity but on occasion is quite copious. In bitches which have been mated there is some difference of opinion as to whether this discharge may not reflect the existence of a pregnancy initially.

Late onset behavioural symptoms

Subjects in this category show mainly behavioural signs which are not usually seen until the 56th–63rd day post-oestrus and sometimes even later. The bitch behaves as though about to whelp with restlessness, unwillingness to go out and, in particular, bed-making. Some even seek solitude in an appropriate place and if carefully observed will make apparent weak straining efforts. This may be followed by a change to nursing behaviour, the bitch taking objects into her bed and huddling around them in a typical mothering posture. In some patients evidence of maternal behaviour is the first sign. Psychological distress occurs frequently. Lactation may or may not occur.

Treatment

Treatment of this type of case comprises several approaches which should be adapted to the main manifestations.

Hormonal

The use of a short, sharp course of oestrogen is often very effective, e.g. 2–5 mg stilboestrol by mouth (according to size) twice daily for 4 or at the most 5 successive days. If this dosage is maintained for a longer time signs of oestrus, e.g. vulval swelling, may occur. Doses lower than this are likely to be ineffective but it is probably wiser not to exceed 10 mg daily even in very large bitches.

Important Note to Readers: At an advanced stage in publication it has been learned that an appeal to the E.E.C. authorities to exempt small animals from the ban on the distribution of stilboestrol for veterinary use has failed. Stilboestrol will, therefore, not be available to veterinary clinicians working within the ambit of the Community. Wherever in the text stilboestrol has been recommended, another agent with oestrogenic activity, such as oestradiol, will have to be substituted in clinical use.

Sedation

If the bitch is sufficiently distressed sedation is called for. Ataractics are not indicated. The very old-fashioned mixture containing potassium bromide and syrup of chloral is usually remarkably effective.

Management

Contrary to what most owners instinctively do, signs of maternal behaviour should be discouraged, e.g. bedding should not be provided, access to the selected 'whelping' area should be prevented or restricted and the nursing of inanimate objects discouraged. Food intake should be reduced to a minimal maintenance ration and, if lactation is present, fluids should be restricted. The bitch should be vigorously encouraged to take exercise and interesting activities outside the home should be increased.

Lactating bitches

It may be arguable as to whether categories 2 and 3 should be divided, but some subjects in category 2 do not lactate and some in category 3 do not display a pesudo-parturient phase. The signs of lactation are obvious and in some patients milk production is so copious that milk drips from the teats. There is some breed variation in this category and most clinicians would agree that dachshunds lactate par excellence!

Treatment

This meets with variable success. Oestrogen, as suggested above, is very effective in many patients and can be repeatedly used at metoestrous periods; in general most bitches respond satisfactorily and milk production ceases within about 7 days. Refractory cases pose a considerable problem and no regularly successful line of treatment for these exists. Obviously reduction in food and drink intake is necessary.

Some bitches are self-suckers and it is essential to emphasize to owners that this must be prevented; that versatile garment, the Baby-gro, can be most useful in this respect. Severe and generalized mastitis has been seen in self-sucking bitches and has even occasionally necessitated total mastectomy, infection presumably being introduced via the teats.

At the best repeated episodes of lactation may result in the failure of mammary tissue and overlying skin to regress after milk production stops. This is not only unsightly but can cause positive problems as in the case of one dachshund bitch which actually stood on and tripped over her own mammae — plastic surgery of a 'face-lift' type was needed. On the other hand bitches lactating in false pregnancy can make very satisfactory foster mothers provided the introduction of the whelps is carefully supervised. There is no apparent contra-indication to this type of fostering.

Hormonal treatment of false pregnancy

Increased understanding of the complexity of hormonal changes occurring in the bitch throughout oestrus, metoestrus and into anoestrus, that is, the period of false pregnancy illuminates the difficulty often experienced in effecting control by the administration of hormones either orally or systemically.

Clearly the treatments with *oestrogens* and *testosterone* which have sometimes proved successful can in no way be considered either logical or specific, except possibly for extremely limited periods within the false pregnancy phase.

More logical therapies recently suggested have so far met with equally limited success in the treatment of false pregnancy, although relief of specific symptoms may be achieved. This also is not surprising in view of the probable complexity of aetiology of some symptoms. Prostaglandins used for their luteolytic effect have been found considerably less satisfactory in the bitch than in other species, and their routine utilization is not yet recommended by manufacturers of proprietary formulations of the drug. The exhibition of toxic symptoms associated with smooth muscle contractile effects is apparently common in the bitch, but may be minimized by protracted administration over a 72-hour period. However, the developing corpus luteum of the early metoestrous phase is considered relatively resistant to luteolysins so that the effect of treatment may be only partial and transient. The use of luteolysins later in metoestrus during the phase of luteal maturity may, by analogy with their effectiveness upon the corpora lutea of pregnancy, be considered to have an increased likelihood of success, but luteolysis induced at this time is likely only to bring forward the phase of progesterone decline rather than to pre-empt the phase of progesterone domination as desired. Therapeutic use of antiprolactins in specific treatment of the lactational symptoms of false pregnancy has also been reported but with mixed enthusiasm. The drug *bromocriptine,* used in uncontrolled trials on a small number of cases, has been reported of low efficacy, having also a tendency to provoke symptoms of toxic side-effect. In other hands these toxic side-effects have been minimized by the adjustment of the dosage regime and the therapeutic effect has been considered useful.

Neither drug has yet been adequately assessed for its value in this field to be undisputed. This may also be said of the various contraceptive antihormones which may be utilized in the treatment of some troublesome cases, although some successes have been reported. Both *delmadinone acetate* and *megestrol acetate* have been used thus, the former by intramuscular injection at an arbitrary dose rate (2·5–5·0 mg/kg twice at 24-hour intervals) and megestrol orally at 2 mg/kg daily for 5 to 8 days commencing at the onset of symptoms.

In neither case is treatment specifically logical and evidence suggests that it is particularly unwise to spay bitches immediately following suppression of a false pregnancy by this method, since there is a tendency for recurrence of symptoms, in particular lactation.

A more compelling case for the value of *megestrol* and *proligestone* in the context of false pregnancy, though indirectly, is the statistical evidence that bitches treated with these drugs for routine oestrus control exhibit a lower incidence of false pregnancy in subsequent cycles than do others previously untreated. No physiological explanation of this phenomenon is forthcoming and considerable further elucidation of the precise aetiology of various symptoms of the false pregnancy syndrome is necessary before totally logical treatments can be advocated.

Polydipsia

This is not a usual feature of false pregnancy per se in any of the forms described, but its occurrence in the metoestrous period is not uncommon. Increased thirst at this stage of the cycle is an indication for careful investigation as regards pyometra, but perhaps more important, especially in bitches of middle life and above in the diabetes-prone breeds (e.g. miniature and toy poodles, dachshunds, etc.), is the possibility of incipient diabetes mellitus. Glycosuria does not present when hyperglycaemia is below renal threshold, thus serum glucose levels should be investigated. Remission of all suspicious signs usually occurs in anoestrus, and it is therefore essential that cases of polydipsia in metoestrus should be fully evaluated.

Prognosis in all false pregnancy cases

It must be emphasized to owners that the condition will recur after every heat, albeit sometimes in varying degrees, some of the milder cases needing no attention. The suggestion which was made at one time, even by veterinary surgeons, that affected bitches should have one litter has long been recognized as futile by the profession, but not by all owners.

Long-term treatment

Ovarohysterectomy is undoubtedly indicated in severe cases which recur regularly, but is preferably delayed until the subject is over 3 years of age. The effects are most impressive especially in bitches hitherto 'hag-ridden' by their hormones.

Surgery should preferably be done during the anoestrous phase and never when the bitch is lactating. Cases of permanent persistence of milk production after spaying are well recognized, even if uncommon, most of which are refractory to treatment. In subjects in which lactation cannot be suppressed prior to operation the prognosis in this respect should be exceedingly guarded.

Perhaps the only useful information to be deduced from false pregnancy subjects is that they have ovulated, otherwise there could be no luteal phase, and this can be helpful in evaluating an infertility case.

REFERENCES

Concannon P. W. and Hansel W. (1977) Prostaglandins, $F_2\alpha$-induced luteolysis, hypothermia and abortion in beagle bitches. *Prostaglandins* 13, 533-542.

Dore M. A. (1978) The value of vaginal smears in determining ovulation and optimum breeding time in the bitch. *Irish Vet. J.* 32, 54-60.

Evans H. M. and Cole H. H. (1931) *Mem. Univ. Calif.* 9 (2), 65-103.

Frost R. C. (1963) Observations concerning ovarian and related conditions in bitches kept as domestic pets. *Vet. Rec.* 75, 653-654.

Holst P. A. and Phemister R. D. (1975) Temporal sequence of events in the estrous cycle of the bitch. *Am. J. Vet. Res.* 36, 705-706.

Jochle W. and Anderson A. C. (1977) The estrous cycle in the dog: a review. *Theriogenology* 7, 113-140.

Lamming G. E., Foster J. F. and Bulman D. C. (1979) Pharmacological control of reproduction cycles. *Vet. Rec.* 104, 156-160.

Lindsay F. E. F. (1978a) An introduction to endoscopy of the canine bitch post uterine tract. *Pedigree Digest* 5, No. 3, 8-10.

Lindsay F. E. F. (1978b) *Ibid. Pedigree Digest* 5, No. 4, 8-9.

Mann C. J. (1971) Some clinical aspects of problems associated with oestrous and its control. *J. Small Anim. Pract.* 12, 391-397.

Schutte A. P. (1967) Canine vaginal cytology. *J. Small Anim. Pract.* 8, 301-317.

Whitney J. C. (1967) The pathology of the canine genital tract in false pregnancy. *J. Small Anim. Pract.* 8, 247-263.

Withers A. R. and Whitney J. C. (1967) The response of the bitch to treatment with Medroxy progesterone acetate. *J. Small Anim. Pract.* 8, 265-271.

Wright P. J. (1980) The induction of oestrus and ovulation in the bitch using pregnant mare serum gonadotrophin and human chorionic gonadotrophin. *Aust. Vet. J.* 56, 137-140.

Chapter 5

Mating

Because copulation is an essential part of reproduction and is therefore a perfectly natural function, it is too readily assumed by many laymen and some veterinary surgeons that all that is necessary is to put dog and bitch together at something like the right time for a litter to result.

The fact is overlooked that selective breeding, in whatever species, entails the putting together of males and females arbitrarily chosen by the breeder, thus immediately excluding all possibility of natural selection. Whilst domestic dogs seldom pair for life (this is rarely possible) and whilst some bitches and most dogs are promiscuous, in many instances the selected pair are not mutually attracted and mating does not occur unassisted. Libido varies considerably, not only between individuals but to some extent between breeds.

Some description of stud management as practised by most dog breeders may be helpful.

THE MALE

Whenever possible a young dog is introduced to stud work in late puberty or early adult life, this age varying to some extent between breeds and with the physical development of the individual. The advantage of an early start is that sexuality is maximal in the young adult and that his behaviour can be more easily adapted to the requirements of selective breeding. It is, of course, essential to ascertain that the dog has two normally descended testes and that his other external genitalia are anatomically normal and reasonably mature.

The ideal is for the first mate of a novice dog to be an experienced

49

brood bitch which is known to be easy to mate and not too selective in her choice of mate.

The management of potential stud dogs during adolescence is important. Young dogs will mount non-oestrous bitches and other dogs running with them, and as this behaviour can lead to fighting most owners check such sexual advances in their young stock. This is clearly necessary but discretion must be exercised as constant verbal or physical restraint of 'randy' dogs can lead to psychological impotence if it is too severe; it is unreasonable to expect a dog to distinguish between prohibition of behaviour in one circumstance and its encouragement in other, to him similar, circumstances.

It is customary in most breeds for some control to be exercised during the mating and for the bitch to be muzzled or taped, or at least held by the head. Such restraint, though sometimes regarded with disfavour as reducing mating to rape, is in line with general practice in other species where, for example, in the case of thoroughbred horses, even more stringent control is exercised. Whilst stud dogs do not compare in value, their owners nonetheless do not expose them to the risks either of injury by biting or of pain occasioned by misbehaviour of the bitch during the tie, both factors likely to cause subsequent refusal to serve. For similar reasons the amount of courtship permitted is usually limited, dog and bitch either being introduced in adjacent runs or controlled on leads. As the bitch is a spontaneous ovulator sexual arousal prior to service is in no way a requirement for conception, but it is highly desirable that the male should be fully stimulated as it has been shown by Boucher and others (1958) that sexual arousal results in the production of ejaculates of increased sperm density.

Frequently the stud handler controls the hind end of the bitch during mating and it is therefore necessary for the young dog to learn that he is expected to mount a restrained bitch; if he is allowed to serve several experienced bitches which do not need holding he may well refuse to approach the less cooperative, restrained bitch. Although it is customary for some control to be maintained during the tie it is quite unnecessary to do as many breeders do, i.e. try to prevent any movement of the pair; it is probable that some movement is conducive to orgasmal contractions by the bitch ('drawing in' is the breeder's phrase) which may be favourable to sperm transport along the bitch genital tract. Some suggest that once the tie is in operation there is no risk of the bitch misbehaving, but this is not true, as occasionally even an experienced brood bitch may try to roll over after the tie has taken place, so throwing the dog off balance and exerting painful traction on the penis.

For the tie to take place full penetration is essential, i.e. the penis is introduced through the area of the constrictor muscle and the bulb of the penis is held within the vulval labiae. Once penetration has occurred massive penile tumefaction takes place and the constrictor muscle grips the cranial end of the penis; in this way both dog and bitch take an active part. Failure of the constrictor vestibularis to relax during oestrus and the situation regarding non-tie services are described later (p. 57).

Frequency of service

One of the most difficult questions upon which to offer well-founded advice is the frequency with which a dog may be used without long-term or short-term harm.

Stud dogs are expected to mate bitches throughout the year and whilst there are well-recognized spring and autumn peaks for oestrous cycles, there is no long period of rest as would occur in wild canidae. Evidence suggestive of seasonal change in semen composition (Taha et al., 1981) was accompanied by evidence of no seasonal change of libido.

The young dog should not be put into full use until approximately 18 months of age in average breeds. Subsequently the ideal frequency of service would probably be one bitch per fortnight, allowing two to three services per bitch, but as everyone realizes this is simply not practicable. If a dog is used frequently over a 2- to 3-week period he should then have a period of sexual rest of several weeks. There is ample circumstantial evidence that popular dogs used very frequently during their first 2–3 years at stud may develop acquired azoospermia between 3 and 6 years of age; in some cases this is permanent but in others fertility is restored after prolonged rest (e.g. one year or longer). Libido may also be affected. It has also been reported that the collection of ejaculates on a regular basis more frequently than once in 24 or 48 hours may result in a reduced sperm output per ejaculate and the depletion of sperm reserves.

Depending upon the longevity of the breed concerned a good stud dog, not overused in youth, remains fertile into old age. Examples are known of fertility at 13 years in a whippet and 11½ years in a Chow, but it is possibly wise to advise that older dogs still offered at public stud be examined for fertility annually. It is commonly believed that fertility in old dogs is reduced both quantitatively and qualitatively but there is no real evidence to support this view. Obviously the possible effect of drugs such as corticosteroids and anabolic steroids on spermatogenesis must be borne in mind. (Taha et al., 1981b.)

Libido in the male is very variable in degree as is speed of response to an oestrous bitch. Many stud dogs develop a conditioned reflex-type response when certain preparations are made for the mating and are fully aroused by the time they are allowed access to the bitch. To ensure that mating is not solely dependent upon such reflexes some change in mating routine is probably an advantage. It is customary for the bitch to visit the dog, but circumstances do arise when the reverse is preferable and a good stud dog of adequate libido and sound temperament will generally perform equally well 'at home or away'.

Some dogs require a prolonged pre-mating contact time, i.e. living in close proximity to the bitch during pro-oestrus, and some dogs will never mount until the bitch displays overt acceptance behaviour. Very occasionally a dog living with a bitch which he is able to mate will form a permanent bond with her and refuse all others, but this is rare. More frequently dogs are to a lesser extent selective and will mate only a proportion of bitches presented to them.

Whether males of poor libido should be used in a breeding programme is highly debatable. The wisdom of attempting to increase libido by therapeutic means is doubtful, but this is nonetheless regularly requested by breeders. In cases of reduced libido of formerly keen studs general health status should be assessed for likely causative factors such as hypothyroidism or other endocrine disturbance. In young, clinically healthy animals there is no evidence to support the value of routine administration of vitamin E, popularly imagined to increase both libido and fertility. The systemic administration of testosterone and some of its analogues may increase libido, but in immature animals detrimental side-effects due to the acceleration of maturation processes should be considered if stunting due to the premature closure of growth plates is to be avoided.

Increased production of testosterone in vivo can be stimulated by the administration of luteinizing hormone (LH) or testosterone compounds can be administered directly. Testosterone proprionate may be used thus at 2·5 mg twice weekly and the phenylproprionate at up to 10 mg every 14 days.

Some anabolic steroids, particularly oxymetholone and stanozolol, have powerful androgenic side-effects which may provoke noticeably increased libido. They, like all androgens, may cause some depression of spermiogenesis but at therapeutic dose levels this is probably insignificant.

THE FEMALE

The major considerations in the bitch upon which advice is often sought is the age recommended for first mating and the frequency of breeding thereafter. The timing of the first attempt to breed will depend largely on the age at which the bitch reaches puberty, and this varies considerably; there is also some breed difference. Chows are the earliest as judged by the first oestrous cycle which often occurs at 5 months and is seldom delayed beyond 7 months; the average age for the first cycle is 8 to 9 months but in some bitches it is delayed considerably, even up to 2 years being frequently reported. In the latter case advice is often sought as to the desirability and/or feasibility of therapeutic induction of a cycle; this is a debatable subject and can only be decided after full evaluation of all the circumstances but it must be emphasized that to obtain an ovulatory cycle requires great care.

It is now believed that delayed breeding can be a cause of infertility or at least reduced fecundity. Many breeders/exhibitors delay breeding in order to complete a successful show career in a promising individual, often postponing mating until the bitch is 3½ to 4 years of age. In a significant proportion of such cases it has been noted that oestrous cycles which had initially been normal in a given bitch become feebler and the bitch becomes anoestrous at a relatively early age. Attempts to mate such bitches once the heats have become less intense usually fail or are infertile.

Ideally it is probably best to mate a bitch initially at a cycle which occurs between 11 and 18 months of age; it is seldom desirable for a bitch to have the first litter earlier than 13 or 14 months but it has to be admitted that puppies which have bred before 12 months seldom seem to have been adversely affected. The latest age for first mating recommended by the author is 2½ years. Obviously there are many instances of successful first breeding from much older bitches but prolonged observation suggests that such delay carries some risk of unsatisfactory breeding performance.

The desirable frequency of breeding is also debatable. At one time it was believed that it should not be more than at alternate heats, so producing approximately one litter annually in bitches of average cycle interval. However, some modification of this view is now held since it would seem that regular breeding is conducive to a more satisfactory breeding career and there are several circumstances in which a breeding regime of two out of every three cycles can be advised. This periodicity is acceptable if the following criteria are met:

1. The previous litter has not been large for the breed concerned.
2. The bitch has adequately reared her litter without undue loss of condition.
3. The interval between cycles is not less than 6 months. Often the anoestrous phase is several weeks longer than average following a litter.

Expressed in a more positive way, breeding at two successive heats can be confidently recommended following the birth of a smallish litter, if the bitch is in top condition and her next cycle occurs 7 months or more after the previous heat.

Another point upon which veterinary advice is often sought is the age at which a bitch can reasonably have her last litter. There can be no precise criteria upon which to base such a decision, but considerations will include the average longevity of the breed, the ease of previous whelpings, the number of litters the bitch has already had, her mothering behaviour and the interval since the previous litter.

Timing and frequency of mating

Whilst it is argued, irrefutably, that a single service from a fertile dog at the right time is sufficient, it is nonetheless true that inopportune mating is a major cause of infertility. In a free-living compatible pair coitus would take place on average once or twice daily throughout the period of acceptance, which might be as long as 7 days, thus ensuring the presence of adequate viable sperm in the genital tract to fertilize ova whenever these are shed. As always variations are common, one of which is that some pairs mate once only despite freedom of contact; at the other extreme the case was reported of a dog and bitch which mated five times in 24 hours — this, however, is unusual.

It is generally agreed that ovulation in the bitch takes place some 24-72 hours after the onset of oestrus, and whether all follicles rupture simultaneously or whether this is spread over a period of hours or days has been studied by Wildt et al., (1978). There is also evidence that in pubertal bitches the time of ovulation in relation to first acceptance of the dog by the bitch is far more regularly fixed at 24-48 hours than is the case in older bitches. This presumably relates to the increasing willingness of experienced bitches to stand for mating. Formation of polar bodies to complete meiosis occurs in the middle and uterine portions of oviducts some 3 to 5 days after first acceptance. The variability of this time interval, and a protracted ovulation period, probably explains the phenomenon of multiplicity of sires occasionally noted when a bitch has mated to several dogs.

Oocytes can remain viable for at least 6 days as can spermatozoa within the uterine lumen, though it is probably advisable not to place reliance upon this, but rather to assume a viability of approximately 48 hours and to arrange for replenishment of semen at appropriate intervals. There is also a suggestion that compared with some other species relatively large numbers of spermatozoa are required to be present in the bitch in order to ensure fertilization.

A reasonable regime which offers optimum prospects of fertility is a service every 48 hours for as long as acceptance continues and the male is keen. Unfortunately under modern methods of living this pattern is not always feasible, and the following factors are involved: time and distance to the chosen stud, the bitch owner's freedom of time and travel and the willingness of the stud owner to permit several services, this being largely dependent upon the popularity of the male concerned.

Sending bitches away to stay at the stud dog's premises is open to several objections and disadvantages which include lack of staff to look after visiting bitches, effect on bitch behaviour in a strange environment, difficulty in consulting the owner if for any reason the selected dog is not successful and the very occasional fraudulent substitution of dogs if the owner is not present to identify the one selected. The ideal situation is either to select a dog at a reasonable distance or for the owners to stay several days in the locality of the stud; unreasonable though this practice sounds it is not unusually carried out.

It is essential to impress upon bitch owners that if only a limited number of services is feasible, these must, regardless of considerations of personal convenience, be at the most favourable time during oestrus if fertility is to result. Problems are, however, not infrequently encountered even by experienced dog breeders in determining optimum times for some bitches.

As already stated, it is inadvisable to rely upon determination of the day simply on the basis of first detection of pro-oestral bleeding and the application of a fixed formula.

Greater success attends much closer attention to the individual, when the observant owner can often detect tell-tale changes in behavioural pattern and physical characteristics. In multi-dog establishments, even in the absence of a male, attitudes towards kennel mates may provide a useful guide to the bitch's willingness to stand for mating.

In general terms the signs to look for are cessation or reduction of vaginal bleeding, though this is not an invariable feature, some softening of the turgidly swollen vulval lips and a willingness by the bitch to stand for genital investigation and mounting by the dog. This can often be determined by her reaction to gentle perineal stimualtion, elevation and sideways deflection of the tail base with consequent vulval exposure being characteristic. Some bitches react in a similar fashion to gentle stroking along the back from the sacrum to tail base, and in some the tail-turning reflex is accompanied by adoption of an exaggerated standing posture with the perineum thrust upwards. In cases of doubt, particularly in bitches showing less or more than the usual discharge of 'colour', the technique of vaginal cytology can be useful.

Some stud dogs show a marked preference to serve bitches early or late in the oestrous phase and it may be necessary to take this into account.

THE TIE

Whilst it is clearly more satisfactory if the so-called tie takes place it is well known that non-tie services are often fertile. The duration of the tie varies from 5 to 45 minutes. Very prolonged ties have been reported — one of 3 hours with a fatal outcome to the dog despite veterinary assistance. An increasing length of tie has also been noted in an ageing dog, possibly indicating some interference with venous drainage from the tumefied penis.

Dog semen comprises three fractions and the success of non-tie services is dependent upon sufficiently persistent duration of penetration to allow ejaculation of the second fraction. The first fraction, probably from the urethral mucous glands, is ejaculated early in normal matings, probably during preliminary thrusting and penetration but certainly immediately after intromission. This fraction is watery and contains no sperm, with a volume of 0·25-2·0 ml. It often has a characteristic odour. The second is the sperm-bearing fraction and is of variable opacity but should not be clear, having a volume of 0·5-3·5 ml. The latent phase between penetration and erection and the ejaculation of the second fraction is variable between individuals and is the vital factor in a dog's ability to fertilize from a non-tie service. In some dogs the second fraction is ejaculated almost simultaneously with complete penetration but in others there is an interval of 30-90 seconds before the sperm is delivered. Hence some dogs will fertilize bitches if penetration persists only briefly; in others it is necessary to hold the dog in the mounted position for 2 or 3 minutes to ensure conception. Ejaculation can be monitored by noting the pulsation of the accelerator urinae muscle in the perineum and this is also shown by a rhythmic movement of the dog's tail. The third fraction comprising prostatic fluid is of volume varying from 2 to 30 ml. According to the results of Wheaton et al. (1979) this volume is proportional to the size of the prostate gland whether normal or benignly hyperplastic. Ejaculation of this fraction continues intermittently throughout the tie. Although prostatic fluid is concerned with sperm transport it is not necessary for fertilization. In matings where large volumes of prostatic fluid are ejaculated there is usually some overflow of fluid from the vagina at the completion of the tie. Owners are sometimes worried that the ejaculate may not have been retained and that the service is therefore unsuccessful.

SOME OBSTACLES TO SUCCESSFUL COITION

Males

Psychological impotence has already been mentioned, and poor libido and slow arousal are other factors which may prevent successful coition. Behavioural aberrations include abnormal mounting position, the dog being willing to mount everywhere except the right place. Some dogs show an initial reluctance to get near enough to the bitch during pelvic thrusting, but once a successful mating has been experienced the problem usually resolves itself. In these circumstances it may be legitimate to use chorionic gonadotrophin to stimulate libido and achieve an initial success. Dogs with high libido can become overstimulated whilst waiting to serve a bitch and become less efficient as a result. Premature ejaculation has also been reported.

Physical discomfort is sometimes seen in dogs with active lesions of dog-pox or other lesions of the penis or prepuce. Contusion of the penile tip may also cause problems, particularly of haemorrhage following mating. In one case encountered in a well-used stud dog, progress of healing was very slow but there was an eventual response to local injection of corticosteroids and antibiotics. In other cases success has followed surgical resection of damaged tissue followed by a period of sexual abstinence.

Persistence of the penile frenulum, like phimosis, obviously precludes service, but both conditions usually cause clinical signs at puberty and are dealt with at that stage.

Females

Abnormalities of the vagina which prevent or interfere with penetration have already been mentioned (p. 23). The commonest cause of vaginal obstruction to intromission is failure of the constrictor vestibularis muscle to relax during oestrus. This is fairly common and is sometimes associated with poor libido; however it has been met in bitches which show normal acceptance behaviour. On digital examination the closed or partially closed muscle prevents access to the vagina proper. Pressure on the area causes marked discomfort to the bitch. Sometimes the structure feels almost membranous, a small central aperture having sensitive, paper-thin edges. This is often described by breeders as a stricture or is thought to be a hymen. It is common practice with some breeders to undertake a crude digital exploration, known as 'breaking the bitch down', prior to attempted mating.

The vast majority of such cases respond extremely well to the use of ataractics; chlorpromazine is often the drug of choice owing to its action on smooth muscle. Dosage is one-half to two-thirds of the normally computed dose; relaxation occurs in most bitches in 20–30 minutes but may take a little longer. Mating can usually be achieved easily at this stage at which time sedation is not marked and the bitch can stand without difficulty; a normal tie is usual.

In a lesser number of cases the vulva remains somewhat prepubertal in type, the upper commissure does not enlarge and soften during oestrus and hence penetration is difficult, painful and often impossible. Ataractics have a much less marked effect than in the previous condition.

Müllerian duct remnants are identified by digital examination and create a variable degree of obstruction to mating.

ARTIFICIAL INSEMINATION

Artificial insemination is used routinely in many countries, both to avoid some of the problems of difficult matings and to utilize imported semen.

The British Kennel Club will not permit the registration of progeny resulting from artificial insemination of a bitch unless prior permission has been obtained and the operation is carried out under strictly controlled conditions which include the presence of a veterinary surgeon. It must be emphasized that Kennel Club permission is granted only in the most exceptional circumstances.

These strictures do not, however, apply to the registration of artificial insemination progeny by many foreign kennel clubs, and it seems likely that because of its obvious advantages, the popularity of the practice will increase. Although no certification is required for semen export from this country, varying health certification relevant to the donor is usually required by the importing country. Certification is usually based on routine clinical examination, often including a blood test for leptospirosis, performed within 14 days of export. With this in mind it is advisable to refrain from vaccinal booster injections of the donor prior to collection of semen for export.

The collection of semen is a relatively straightforward procedure but the techniques of semen evaluation, dilution and deep-freeze storage are not and it is advisable that supervision of these techniques be in the hands of specialists.

Semen Collection

Semen collection from the conscious dog is performed most efficiently in the presence of a 'teaser' oestrous bitch, although some experienced stud dogs require no such stimulation. Conversely some studs are unwilling to submit to manipulation and defy all attempts at semen collection.

Harrop (1954) has described the design of a pulsatile artificial vagina as occasionally useful even in the absence of a 'teaser' bitch, but the commoner collection technique is by digital manipulation of the penis. This requires firm grasping of the extruded shaft of the semi-erect penis behind the bulbus glandis, where the application of gentle pressure induces coital thrusting movements and ejaculation. By this means it is usually possible to collect the three fractions of ejaculate separately. In some dogs which are slow to respond a combined massaging action behind the bulbus may obtain erection and ejaculation. A good deal of patience is needed in some subjects and attempts to collect should not be abandoned too easily.

Semen evaluation

This is performed routinely before its deep-freeze storage or use for artificial insemination. This examination, as in a fertility test, is for motility, sperm density and morphology. A simple examination for sperm density and motility can easily be performed in practice, bearing in mind two points:

1. Canine sperm is speedily immobilized by contact with rubber and latex, hence this should not be used in collection apparatus or a false diagnosis of poor motility may be made.

2. The wave motion characteristic of bovine semen is not seen in dog sperm in which random, rapid, darting movement is more typical (see p. 172).

Artificial insemination of the bitch, either with freshly collected or stored semen, depends for its success as much on assessment of the stage of oestrus of the bitch as on the dexterity of the inseminator. This assessment may be based on visible external signs and the bitch's willingness to stand for mounting, or on vaginal cytological examination. In either event, as in normal service, insemination on two occasions at 24- to 48-hour intervals is recommended.

Relatively makeshift equipment can be utilized for insemination, the main requirement being a catheter or pipette of adequate length and diameter to be used alone or in conjunction with a vaginal speculum.

The bitch, with external genitalia suitably cleansed, is restrained with her hind end slightly elevated and the speculum is introduced as far as the cervix, allowing placement of the tip of the catheter through or close to the cervix. Norwegian specialists, using specially designed cannulae, claim intra-uterine insemination to be invariably possible, but it seems unlikely on the basis of the results of others that such precise placement is critical for the achievement of conception.

Semen introduced via the cannula may be gravity fed or forced gently by syringe pressure and the bitch should remain with hindquarters slightly elevated for a few moments after withdrawal to prevent undue loss by abrupt change of posture. Introduction of a finger into the vagina immediately after the cannula is removed can achieve two objectives: plugging of the vagina to minimize spillage of semen and, if gentle massaging movements are made, the stimulation in some bitches of the rhythmic contractions, often seen during a natural tie, which assist semen transport. Owners should not be encouraged to do this unless they are adequately trained in cleanliness of method.

In some cases tranquillization or anaesthesia of the recipient may be necessary to permit insemination and surgical intra-uterine insemination may also be performed. Inadequate data are available on which to base relative assessment of these techniques, but it is emphasized that the timing and placement of stored semen is more critical than that of fresh semen, presumably because many spermatozoa are rendered incapable of penetrating ova as a consequence of freezing.

The preparation of semen for short- or long-term storage and transit requires clean collection of the sperm-bearing second fraction ejaculate. After examination for viability this is diluted to standard sperm density for storage. For short-term storage and transport at $4°C$ a simple milk diluent is satisfactory. Pasteurized milk, maintained at $92-94°C$ for 10 minutes then cooled to room temperature, is used to dilute semen, usually in the ratio of approximately 8 : 1, prior to cooling for storage at $4°C$. Suitably protected vials of the dilute can be maintained at this temperature during transit by being packed in crushed ice in simple vacuum flasks, and viability of several days' duration is recorded.

For long-term deep-freeze storage and more distant transit a diluent of egg yolk, sodium citrate buffer with glycerol is preferred. The dilute is taken up into straws and refrigerator-cooled for several hours before reduction to $-196°C$, the temperature of liquid nitrogen under which straws are stored. Critical evaluation of the success of freezing is based on post-thaw motility which usually varies from 20 to 90%, 50 to 70% being regarded as satisfactory. The semen of some individuals may fail to freeze satisfactorily, but most problems are apparently attributable to the egg yolk component of the diluent.

Many well-authenticated reports of the long-term viability of correctly frozen and stored canine semen have now been recorded. Conception rates under laboratory conditions may be as high as 70%, but field results are lower, though improved by repeat inseminations. Practical evidence suggests that dilution of semen to the degree practised in cattle AI is not feasible, one or more whole ejaculates being required to ensure a reasonable chance of conception.

The litters born following freeze-storage of semen tend to be smaller than usual for the breed concerned, although large litters have been achieved. The reason for this remains unknown.

REFERENCES

Boucher, J. H., Foote R. H. and Kirk R. W. (1958) The evaluation of semen quality in the dog and the effects of frequency of ejaculation upon semen quality, libido and depletion of sperm reserves. *Cornell Vet.* 48, 67–86.

Harrop A. E. (1954) A new type of canine artificial vagina. *Br. Vet. J.* 110, 194–196.

Jochle W. and Anderson A. C. (1977) The estrous cycle in the dog: a review. *Theriogenology* 7, 113–140.

Morton D. B. (1980) *Details of artificial insemination technique.* Personal communication. University of Leicester, England.

Taha M. B., Noakes, D. E. and Allen W. E. (1981a) The effect of season of the year on the characteristics and composition of dog semen. *J. Small Anim. Pract.* 22, 177–184.

Taha M. B., Noakes D. E. and Allen W. E. (1981b) The effect of some exogenous hormones on seminal characteristics, libido and peripheral plasma testosterone concentration in the male beagle. *J. Small Anim. Pract.* 22, 589–595.

Wheaton L. G., DeKlerk D. P., Strandberg J. D. et al. (1979) Relationship of seminal volume to size and disease of the prostate gland in the beagle. *Am. J. Vet. Res.* 40, 1325–1328.

Wildt D. E., Chakraborty P. K., Panko W. B. and Seager S. W. J. (1978) Relationship of reproductive behaviour, serum luteinizing hormone and time of ovulation in the bitch. *Biol. Reprod.* 18, 561–570.

FURTHER READING

Grandage J. (1972) The erect dog penis: a paradox of flexible rigidity. *Vet. Rec.* 91, 141–147.

Chapter 6

Pregnancy

DURATION

Whilst the gestation period for the bitch is always quoted as 63 days all veterinary surgeons are only too well aware of the variations. Probably 56 to 70 days could be taken as the extreme limits of normality; whelps born from the 56th day onwards are usually viable, always assuming that there is no pathological reason for fetal death, but those born prior to the 56th day seldom survive, solely due to immaturity. It is an interesting observation that whelps born several days before term are usually well within normal limits for size and maturity. There is some difficulty in deciding at what stage the persistence of gestation beyond 63 days becomes abnormal; there are numerous authenticated instances of apparently normal whelping up to and on the 70th day, nonetheless there is always anxiety in such cases.

Some people, owners and veterinary surgeons alike, prefer the regime of a single service so that the date of anticipated parturition is accurately known. However, the duration of pregnancy will not necessarily depend upon the date of mating as it is related to the time of fertilization. This, in its turn, is dependent upon the simultaneous presence of fertilizable ova and viable sperm in the oviducts which can be subject to a variation of up to 48 hours, hence objections to a multiple-service system are probably not valid. In practice the date of whelping has always been estimated from the date of first service.

PREGNANCY DIAGNOSIS

Palpation of fetal units

Tubal travel and nidation

The period of transit of fertilized ova along the Fallopian tubes is long, i.e.

8 days, and nidation occurs at 16 days at the earliest. Examination of the genital tracts of bitches in early pregnancy shows clearly that the fertilized units tend to distribute themselves evenly along the two uterine horns so that there is no great disparity between the horns, e.g. one ovary may show five corpora lutea and the other only two but the conceptuses are almost certain to be divided four and three.

The long interval between mating and nidation accounts for the success of oestrogens in preventing pregnancy in cases of misalliance. Once the endometrium is returned to the state of being under oestrogen control it is inimical to implantation, hence injections given as long as 4 days after an unwanted mating are nearly always successful.

Development of fetal units

From 18 days onwards firm spherical enlargements develop at each nidation site; at 21 days each fetal unit is often described as being the size of a pea, some 0·75–1·0 cm in diameter. Many veterinary surgeons prefer to undertake pregnancy diagnosis by palpation at this stage and in small relaxed subjects it is very successful; in larger bitches with substantial abdominal tissues it is far from easy (*Fig. 3*).

By 28 days the units have reached 2·5–3·5 cm in diameter with a length of only slightly enlarged uterine horn between each unit. Many veterinarians believe this to be the optimum stage for diagnosis by palpation which can be achieved in a high proportion of bitches between the 26th and 31st

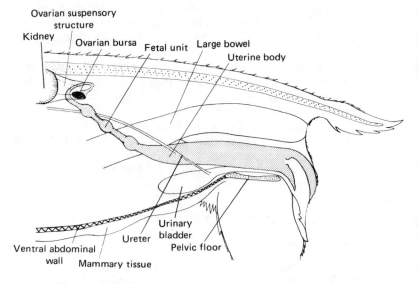

Fig. 3. Approximately 21-day pregnancy with pea-sized fetal units.

days. It is essential to emphasize to owners the need for this examination to take place within these narrow limits since, not unreasonably, they assume that the later it takes place the better as the conceptuses will be larger and thus more easily felt (*Fig. 4*).

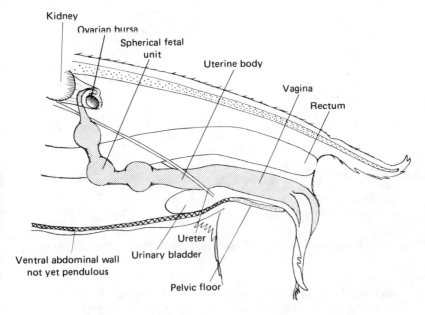

Fig. 4. Approximately 28-day pregnancy with palpable fetal units sagging toward abdominal floor.

The range of size of 28-day-old fetal units is surprisingly small considering the very big size variation between breeds, e.g. the fetal unit of a Newfoundland is not twelve times larger than that of a Pekingese.

After 30 days accumulation of fetal fluids results in the units enlarging more rapidly, losing the tense feel and becoming ovoid in shape. The uterine horn between units becomes larger and softer hence palpation becomes more difficult, almost impossible, in all but very relaxed, thinly muscled bitches (*Fig. 5*).

Precise recognition of the gravid uterus is often not possible after 30 days until ossification of the fetal head renders it again palpable at about 49 days, by which time pregnancy may be obvious.

Diagnosis by means other than palpation

Biological tests appear to remain unreliable in the bitch. In view of the susceptibility of embryonic tissue to radiation radiography cannot be

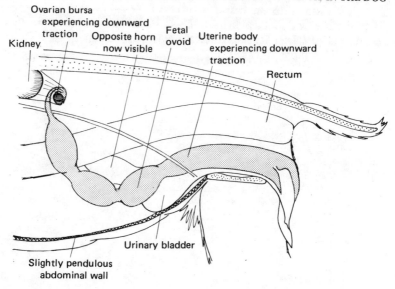

Fig. 5. Approximately 35-day pregnancy with fetal ovoids difficult to palpate.

commended for routine use solely for pregnancy diagnosis, other than at or after term when doubts exist as to the presence of fetuses.

The following are some of the objective signs which may be shown by pregnant bitches.

Teats

These show enlargement, erectility, reddening (mainly in light-skinned subjects) and occasionally development of an areolar area. These signs become apparent from 28 days onwards and are more obvious in primigravidae.

Mammary tissue

The onset of development of active mammary tissue is very variable, from about 35 days to just before term. It is not always easy to differentiate from the mammary hyperplasia of false pregnancy. Likewise the start of milk production and let-down is exceedingly variable from 49 days (one bitch is known to have actually suckled a puppy from another dam at this stage) until after the completion of whelping. Marked preparturient waxing of the teats has been seen in one subject.

Vaginal discharge

This is probably the most reliable indication of pregnancy other than palpation. A mucoid very viscid secretion is noticed at the vulva usually from approximately 32 days until shortly before term. A bitch showing no such discharge is unlikely to be pregnant. The quantity varies from a copious discharge hanging in strings from the vulva, to a mere stickiness of the hair around the vulva. A similar discharge commencing as late as 42 to 49 days is more likely to signal the end of a false pregnancy.

Changes in behaviour

These are only suggestive, but observant owners can be reasonably accurate in the interpretation of some features. Many pregnant bitches show no change in temperament and behaviour and remain active until and unless gross abdominal enlargement develops. Lethargy and early abdominal enlargement are more likely to indicate false pregnancy.

Some nervous bitches become more tranquil and affectionate. Whilst appetite is increased in many subjects there are many in which a considerable degree of anorexia occurs, usually between 30 and 56 days; surprisingly, whelps from such bitches show no evidence of the dam's inappetence. Many bitches refuse milk even if they have previously liked it.

There is occasionally increased desire for water in mid-pregnancy which can be a cause for concern if there is no history of mating and a loculated uterus can be palpated. Vigorous scratching of the ventral body surface along the mammary area is seen in many pregnant bitches but seldom in false pregnancies, even if lactation occurs; this may start as early as the 28th day.

Abdominal distension is not a reliable feature. Possibly the most significant change is in bitches pregnant with multiple fetuses when folding of the uterine horns occurs at about 42 days resulting in a relatively sudden drop in the outline of the abdomen (*Fig.* 6).

Fetal movements can be felt and occasionally seen in heavily gravid bitches during the last 7 days but by this time other signs of pregnancy are usually obvious (*Fig.* 7).

Failure to diagnose pregnancy at or near term can occasionally result in claims of negligence in this increasingly litigious age, and it is at this stage that radiography should be utilized as a diagnostic measure. There can be little excuse for not invoking this aid in cases of doubt, and if owners demur or refuse on grounds of radiation hazard responsibility for the decision must unequivocally be laid on their shoulders, preferably in the presence of a witness. The more sophisticated technique of ultrasonic fetometry might also be applicable in such circumstances, its advantage over radiological examination being provision of proof of fetal life by the measurement of heart rate and the detection of characteristic sounds of

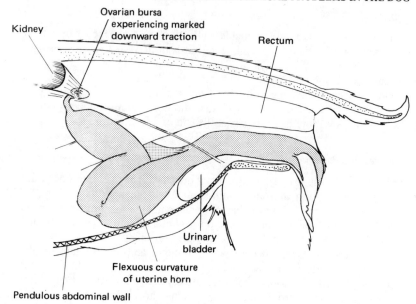

Fig. 6. Approximately 42-day pregnancy with folding of uterine horn to accommodate fetal unit.

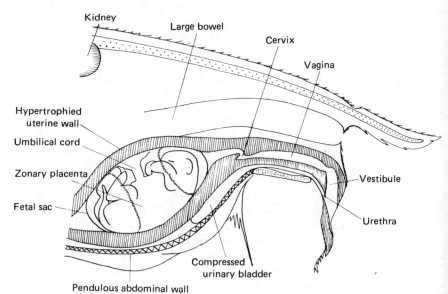

Fig. 7. Sagittal section of uterine horn to exhibit typical alignment of a late fetal unit.

placental circulation. Ultrasonic equipment is, of course, less readily available than straightforward radiography, but the advantages of its use, particularly in the assessment of continuing progress of a doubtful pregnancy, have recently been reported by Jackson and Nicholson (1979) and reviewed by Allen and Meredith (1981).

COMPLICATIONS OF PREGNANCY

Resorption, abortion and premature parturition

The premature termination of gestation by resorption of whole litters or abortion of live or dead fetuses is relatively uncommon in the bitch.

There is clear evidence that resorption on a limited scale does occur. It is neither uncommon for fewer whelps to be delivered at full term than were palpable in utero at 28 days, nor is it unusual during Caesarean hysterotomy to note sites of limited placental development at which resorption has occurred. In the majority of such cases it is likely that primary aetiological factors are uterine overcrowding or premature fetal death due to a combination of lethal genetic factors, and there is no evidence of intra-uterine disease or infertility. Occasionally during the investigation of infertility there is a suggestion that resorption of whole litters has occurred in individual cases, but usually this is based on circumstantial rather than definite evidence of conception.

Abortion of identifiable fetuses in late pregnancy takes several forms and is occasionally more properly considered as premature parturition. Some bitches habitually whelp early and produce viable whelps after gestation periods of little over 56 days. Others, after an only slightly shorter gestation period, produce live but non-viable whelps. In these latter cases it is assumed that premature parturition is the result of primary endocrinological changes and though hormone profiles are not available, premature withdrawal of progesterone is postulated, with the cause of luteolysis unknown. Since it is arguable whether bitch or fetus provides the trigger to parturition, it is usually recommended that the bitch be subsequently put in whelp to a different dog in order to ensure a fresh combination of genes in the resultant fetuses. Under field conditions it is regrettably often impossible to evaluate the success of this policy in individual cases, but in support of the thesis of fetal responsibility, it is interesting to note that owners of stud dogs occasionally remark upon the tendency of some dogs to sire puppies almost invariably carried a full 63 days' gestation or longer out of a variety of bitches. In some cases, however, accumulated evidence apparently indicates the endocrinological failure to occur within the bitch, the cause of premature loss of luteal function remaining obscure but presumably relating to the withdrawal of luteotropic support of pituitary or even placental origin.

Fetal losses in some bitches occur at times or in circumstances so removed from parturition that they must realistically be classified as abortion. In these cases part or whole litters of non-viable or dead puppies are produced in a variety of circumstances. Veterinary literature contains numerous records detailing premature onset of parturition with loss of blood and tissue and one or several whelps, but subsequent delivery at full term of normal viable puppies. In these cases the cause of death of individual fetal units is usually enigmatic and the retention and subsequent delivery of live puppies is occasionally attributed to various hormonal treatments administered, although equally satisfactory results may follow simple antibiotic therapy or even no treatment. In some cases abortion is threatened rather than actual, the bitch eventually producing, among the normal whelps at term, a dead fetus presenting signs of earlier placental detachment and loss of blood and fetal fluids.

Symptoms suggestive of impending fetal loss most frequently occur at between 6 and 7 weeks of gestation, often initially as bloodstained vulval discharge. Confusingly, such blood loss is occasionally unassociated with intra-uterine changes, rather being attributable to vaginal lesions, often apparently located in the region of the urinary meatus and hypothesized to result from mating trauma. Because of the possibility of so relatively harmless an aetiology of haemorrhagic vulval discharge, and because of the potentially fetotoxic and complicating effects of gross hormonal therapy aimed at abortion prevention, it is advisable that in the first instance investigation and treatment be cautiously instituted. Thus, after careful digital or endoscopic examination of the vagina, a haemorrhagic focus may be identified and locally treated, avoiding the unnecessary usage of systemic therapy. In the event of confirmation of impending abortion, vaginal microbiological swabbing is worthwhile so that appropriate antibiotic therapy can be instituted, but apart from this no specific treatment can be recommended. It is possibly preferable to accept the inevitable rather than to administer systemically gross quantities of progesterone hormone which may disadvantageously block progress of cervical dilatation and uterine evacuation and which are unlikely to exercise useful abortion-averting effects without placing fetal life at risk.

Infection

The loss of entire litters of dead and occasionally autolysing fetuses and membranes in circumstances suggestive of intra-uterine infection rather than endocrinological disturbance does occasionally occur, with the apparent involvement of a variety of aetiological factors. However, in marked contrast with other species, there are few authenticated records of 'abortion storms' even among closely kennelled bitches, regardless of the infections implicated. The potential of *Brucella abortus* infection to provoke such a situation is suggested by a circumstantial report of the abortions of two infected bitches on the same premises within a 6-week period, but against this the failure of other exposed kennel mates to contract the infection apparently indicates a relative canine resistance to the disease. This infection, encountered in scavenging bitches having access to uncooked bovine tissues and discharges, is associated with the appearance of purulent vaginal discharge early in pregnancy, with abortion occurring around the 50th day of gestation and the subsequent discharge of organisms taking place over a variable, occasionally prolonged period. However, the frequency with which many bitches had access to *Br. abortus*-infected tissues when this organism was common in the national herd is in marked contrast to the rarity of even suspected cases of clinical infection in the dog. Under present conditions it would be extremely rare to make a putative, let alone confirmed, diagnosis of *Br. abortus* as a cause of abortion in the bitch.

Not yet endemic to this country is *Br. canis* which is reported to be involved in cases of abortion and infertility, especially on a kennel basis, in the United States of America. Since antibodies to the infection have already been isolated from imported breeding stock it is inevitable that the disease will eventually be recognized here.

As described it is characterized by a reduced pup yield variously attributable to conception failures, resorption and abortion, with transmission by contact with infected discharges and venereally. Even in large kennel units disease may be encountered on a fairly limited basis with infected animals identifiable serologically by tube agglutination tests. A policy of isolation and eradication is advocated.

Abortion in association with virally induced systemic disease may occasionally be encountered, but specifically abortifacient viruses are few in number. In this category, canine herpes virus, though more commonly associated with neonatal puppy losses, has been identified by inclusion bodies within areas of placental degeneration and necrosis and may be assumed thus to be responsible for abortion in some cases.

Teratogens

Non-infective aetiological factors resulting in abortion secondary to fetal damage or death may be encountered without identification. These may often pass unremarked unless dramatically presented as, for instance, on a kennel basis. In this category are such various factors as heat stress and exposure to teratogens.

The effects of sustained hyperthermia in several non-canine species have been reported as ovulatory failure, embryonic mortality, disturbed prenatal development, low birth weight and prematurity. It is interesting to speculate how far towards this situation kennel management habits may be progressing. It is also noteworthy that during the hot summer of 1974 some stud dog owners reported a higher than usual number of infertile matings followed by a return to fertility at the following cycle in many cases.

The exposure of pregnant bitches to previously unimagined teratogens, usually accidentally contracted as crop sprays, etc, has resulted in the birth of entire litters conspicuously affected by non-lethal developmental defects. It is therefore not difficult to visualize circumstances in which directly ecbolic effects of such chemicals, or their lethal teratogenic effects, might result in abortion. Since the teratogenic effects of individual agents depend precisely upon the stage of fetal development at the time of exposure, it must be anticipated that the clinical response to random exposure will vary.

Tubal pregnancy and ectopic pregnancy

These have occasionally been reported in other species and presumably may occur in the bitch. Both conditions would be likely to present as abdominal emergencies without specific symptomatic reference to the reproductive tract.

Torsion of the uterus

Although this complication of late pregnancy has been regularly reported in the cat, its occurrence in the bitch is extremely rare. The suggestion that this condition might be aetiological in occasional unsuspected mummification of fetuses in utero is difficult to substantiate. Certainly, one well-authenticated case of torsion did occur during the last few days of pregnancy and presented as an abdominal catastrophe with profound shock. The bitch failed to survive the laparotomy at which precise diagnosis was made, and it seems likely that most cases would have a similarly unsatisfactory outcome.

It is difficult to visualize the likelihood of torsion in bicornuate or multi-fetal pregnancies, but as a precautionary measure it is probably advisable to restrain heavily gravid bitches from excessive play or rolling behaviour.

REFERENCES

Allen W. E. and Meredith M. J. (1981) Detection of pregnancy in the bitch: a study of abdominal palpation, A-mode ultrasound and Doppler ultrasound techniques. *J. Small Anim. Pract.* 22, 609–622.
Jackson P. G. G. and Nicholson J. M. (1979) The use of ultrasound to monitor fetal life in a pregnant bitch. *Vet. Rec.* 104, 36.

Chapter 7

Normal Whelping

Parturition in the bitch is traditionally described, as in other species, in the classical three stages, namely:

First stage: Progressive relaxation and dilatation of the cervix instigated by intra-uterine fluid pressure.

Second stage: Delivery of the fetuses. This should commence when the cervix is fully dilated.

Third stage: Expulsion of the fetal membranes which, in multi-fetal species having individual placentae, is repeated in a variable pattern between births.

FIRST-STAGE LABOUR

This is extremely variable in several respects in the bitch. Basically it represents the phase of preparation for the birth and is thus largely seen by way of behavioural signs. Although many bitches undoubtedly experience some discomfort it is not essentially a painful period. An unusual degree of pain has been seen in late first-stage labour on a few occasions when uterine contractions have become powerful before full relaxation of the cervix has occurred.

Duration

This is immensely variable from none being observable to 48 hours, but it is arguable whether the latter figure is not verging on abnormality; the average is 6 to 20 hours. The nil duration suggested above is the situation in which the bitch has shown no sign whatsoever of impending parturition (no temperature checking undertaken), is often taken for a walk and drops the first pup without warning. This state of affairs has been noted on a number

71

of occasions and will be familiar to most clinicians, but it is unusual. One such case was that of a Poodle under the close supervision of an exceedingly competent and experienced veterinary practitioner, so these are not examples of faulty observation as might be assumed.

Variations in length of the first stage depend upon several factors, some of which are described below:

Temperament

Placid bitches with good maternal behaviour are less likely to have a protracted first stage. Neurotic household pets in which natural instincts have been largely sublimated in their attachment to owners are prone to long first-stage labour and even hysterical behaviour; in extreme cases the use of modest doses of ataractic drugs is effective and well justified (e.g. Chlorpromazine hydrochloride B.P. Vet. or acepromazine maleate B.P.C. dosed orally at 1·0 mg/kg, or to effect).

Management

It would be normal for non-domesticated canidae to dig a den at the end of a burrow and there seek seclusion to give birth. Many domestic bitches retain this instinct and attempt to follow it, some successfully, but this is seldom possible; however, not all seek solitude.

Many bitches, mainly those not confined to kennels, show a marked preference for a particular site, usually most unsuitable as judged from the owner's point of view, and are clearly able to delay progress to some extent unless they are allowed their choice. Sites usually selected by owners are not suitable from the bitch's viewpoint as they are seldom under any form of cover.

Whenever possible the bitch should be allowed to whelp in a place acceptable to her and then be transferred to the selected place soon after parturition is completed.

Change of environment is another factor inimical to the smooth progress of first-stage labour. This usually arises in one of two ways:

1. A pet owner, having decided to breed from a bitch, suddenly realizes that a whelping bitch in her usual quarters may be inconvenient and/or messy and decides to consign the animal to the garage or other outside building. Unless the bitch has been habituated to this for *many* weeks prior to whelping there is likely to be a delay in the first stage.

2. Kennel owners sometimes change the bitch's environment by removing her from her usual kennel and bringing her into or nearer the house. Whilst this is done for the best of motives it may cause distress and delay unless the bitch has become used to the new quarters over a long period.

Signs of first-stage labour

The well-recognized signs are restlessness, bed-making, panting and shivering. Abdominal contractions are not seen in this phase except for some rippling of the flanks in the last stages or where there is faulty synchronization as described previously. Intermittent bed-making may be seen for some days prior to whelping and taken on its own is not indicative of first-stage labour.

All the above signs should become progressively more vigorous and continuous throughout the first stage and this point cannot be too strongly emphasized. It is a vital feature to ascertain accurately in history taking. Failure of the signs to escalate in intensity or frequency may be the first hint of uterine inertia. It is highly desirable that inexperienced owners should be accurately informed of the course of normal whelping, either by their veterinary surgeon or by a book recommended by and familiar to the clinician. The author has had a recent experience of a highly qualified nurse who had bred several litters and did not know that the signs described above indicated first-stage labour.

The loss of fetal fluids is very irregular in occurrence and timing and is of little help in evaluating the progress of labour.

Transition from the first to the second stage is difficult to ascertain accurately as it is in part dependent upon the engagement of the fetal head in the birth canal once full dilatation of the cervix has occurred. It can reasonably be said to be longer in some of the brachycephalic breeds, e.g. Pekingese, as firm engagement of the bullet head of the fetus may be somewhat delayed and, in contradiction of what was said earlier, abdominal contractions may be seen in such cases for 1 to 2 hours prior to the onset of regular, meaningful straining. Fortunately in most such breeds size permits a helpful vaginal examination to be made.

It is a helpful routine in practice to encourage owners to advise of the anticipated date of whelping, possibly preceded by pregnancy diagnosis, then to notify the practice when the first stage commences and to report at agreed intervals thereafter. Whilst normal if slow progress can follow even after 36 to 48 hours of first-stage labour, it is probably wise to make a precautionary examination after 24–36 hours unless it is clear that progress is being made. It is also important to instruct owners to report if the signs of first stage become feebler or cease after a few hours. A wait-and-see policy is not advisable.

Owners often seek advice as to the signs of impending parturition, especially if they have to be out for any length of time. Most of the traditional signs suggested in books written by laymen are unreliable. Appetite may or may not be lost, vomiting is unusual and the let-down of milk is no guide. The presence of vaginal discharge prior to whelping, which is so often taken by the layman to be a conclusive sign, is not only misleading but is usually incorrect. The pregnancy discharge usually ceases some days prior to whelping and in most cases no further discharge is seen until the membranes rupture. In a small number of cases, mainly in heavily pregnant bitches, a *light*-green mucoid discharge occurs some 24–48 hours before labour commences.

The most reliable guide is probably the marked but transient drop in rectal temperature. It must be remembered that the temperature of a bitch in the last weeks of pregnancy is below average, e.g. 100°F (37·7°C) and this does not signify impending parturition. Temperature drops in the vast majority of cases to 97–99°F but may persist at this level for only a few hours hence at least twice daily temperature taking is required. First-stage labour should commence within 24 hours of the low temperature being noted and failure to do so should alert suspicions of uterine inertia.

This regime can be especially helpful in bitches pregnant with only one or two fetuses, in which cases the risk of complete primary inertia is well recognized.

SECOND-STAGE LABOUR

The traditional criterion for deciding that second-stage labour has (or should have) commenced is full dilatation of the cervix but, as noted previously, the cervix can only be reached digitally in a small proportion of bitches. It is an unfortunate fact that the constrictor area at the cranial extremity of the vestibule is often mistaken for the cervix.

During the transition from the first to second stage the head or pelvic girdle of the presenting fetus is becoming engaged in the pelvic inlet, and pressure from the engaged part on the cervix stimulates straining efforts, thus contractions of the abdominal mucles are seen. It is important that owners should be made aware that both anterior and posterior presenta-tions are normal for the bitch — it is estimated that some 40% of births are posterior presentations — and that the latter is *not* a breech birth. At the same time it must be recognized that a posteriorly presented puppy can be subject to some delay in one of three ways, especially if it is the first of the litter.

1. Engagement of the soft tissues of the hindquarters provides less stimulus to straining than does the bony skull when engaged in the pelvic inlet.

2. There is occasional hold-up as the pectoral girdle enters the birth canal.

3. Likewise the head may be held up at the pelvic inlet.

These factors will be considered more fully later.

In most cases as second stage supervenes the bitch becomes quieter and more purposeful in behaviour. Fluids are lost intermittently and the bitch repeatedly turns to clean herself; this posture increases intra-abdominal pressure which usually results in several vigorous straining efforts. Subse-quent births are often heralded by a relatively brief return to the more agitated behaviour of the first stage which ceases as soon as the fetus is fully engaged.

Once again there is much variation in the progress of second-stage labour, between both individuals and breeds. The ratio of puppy : dam size is an important factor. When this is wide, as in many of the bigger gundogs which usually have large numbers of puppies, births are usually more rapid both as regards the degree of effort needed to expel a fetus and the interval between deliveries. When the ratio is narrower due to lower litter numbers and the relative size of the fetus, the reverse is true.

There is also a noticeable variation in the vigour of straining and this does not refer to any degree of uterine inertia; there is some breed variation in this respect although this is by no means uniform. Examples which come to mind are the Chihuahua which is often extremely vigorous in its expulsive efforts so that if an obstructive dystocia occurs prompt assistance is essential. Boxers often appear to be doing little or no straining but almost without warning the perineal vagina is seen to be bulging and a puppy slides out apparently without much effort.

In the average case occasional contractions are seen in the early part of second-stage labour. These become more regular, frequent and forceful and usually the final few efforts before the birth are characterized by the bitch arching her back and raising her tail.

The duration of straining before a birth is one of the most difficult points upon which to pontificate and no authoritative statement can be made. The following are suggested as guidelines:

First puppy: This is usually born within one hour of the onset of meaningful straining, but often appears within as little as 20 minutes; up to 2 hours' straining need not cause anxiety. It is probably wise to advise owners to make a telephone report if no puppy is born after 2 hours. By 6 hours placental separation is occurring and the life of the presenting puppy may be in jeopardy, thus 6 hours should be regarded as the maximum period permissible without investigation; even after 2 hours some separation may exist.

Subsequent puppies: The birth canal is now fully dilated thus expulsion should be easier (oversize puppies will be dealt with later), and straining time is usually reduced to 5-30 minutes.

The interval between births is another matter; it comprises two parts — resting and straining. Rest periods vary from 5 minutes to 3 hours and occasionally even longer, although it is arguable if more than 4 hours' rest falls within normal limits. Provided vigorous straining without progress does not occur the longer intervals do not call for urgent attention. A common pattern is for a bitch to produce two or three puppies at short intervals, e.g. 10 to 30 minutes, and then go into a rest phase of 1 to 3 hours before repeating the process.

The birth of a large litter may occupy 24 hours or so but if there is no excessive effort needed for each birth the dam should not become unduly tired.

A bitch with good mothering behaviour will clean and nurse her whelps between successive births and will keep the whelping area clean as well. The desirability of leaving puppies with the bitch during her subsequent labour may be to some extent controversial, but it is the author's belief that this should be done under all normal circumstances.

THIRD-STAGE LABOUR

This is the stage of expulsion of the fetal membranes of which there are two normal variants:

1. The whelp is born enclosed in the intact membranes, the bitch freeing the puppy from them and then separating the cord. Should an inexperienced bitch seem not to know what to do the attendant should tear the membranes and free the head, running a finger through the mouth to remove mucus, at which stage most bitches will take over.

2. The membranes have ruptured and the puppy is not enveloped but is still attached by the umbilical cord. If the bitch severs the cord before the placenta has come out of the vagina it may remain in the vagina or retract into the uterus and be expelled subsequently.

In this latter case the membranes may or may not be expelled before the next birth. In theory it would seem that this must happen but in fact it is quite common for several more births to occur followed by delivery of a batch of sets of membranes, indicating that fetuses are not necessarily delivered alternatively from the two cornua. (van der Weyden et al., 1981).

Whilst it is very helpful if the attendant can correlate the sets of membranes with the eventual number of puppies it cannot always be done as the bitch may eat the placentae with some speed.

There is clearly no need for a domestic bitch to eat the membranes as a source of nourishment immediately postpartum, but it is in no way necessary to interfere with her normal instincts by totally preventing this. It is at least arguable that the placental hormones play a useful part in the subsequent involution and/or milk production.

Many bitches will indicate the termination of whelping by becoming completely relaxed and going to sleep, almost as if with a sigh of relief at a job well done. Owners learn to recognize this but should remember that it is not invariable evidence of completion.

Whether newly whelped bitches should routinely be examined at the apparent termination of whelping is controversial and must be decided by mutual discussion between owner and veterinarian. Believing that a newly whelped bitch is extremely vulnerable to disturbance and stress it is preferable not to make a routine examination unless full discussion with the owner has given any cause for doubt.

Rectal temperature usually rises to 102·5-103°F soon after whelping and this level persists for 2-3 days. This moderate rise should not be taken per se as evidence of postpartum infection.

Owners should be advised that, apart from the examination to determine sex, the presence of hind dewclaws or of any other obvious abnormality, e.g. cleft palate, puppies should be handled as little as possible for the first 2 weeks of life; equally so the number of people allowed to see the dam and litter should be minimal and restricted to those with whom the bitch is fully familiar. The birth of a litter of puppies, whilst an excitement for the family, should never be made a public spectacle as so many people tend to do. Socialization of the puppies is not required until at least 3 weeks of age.

REFERENCE

van der Weyden G. C. et al. (1981) The intra-uterine position of canine foetuses and their sequence of expulsion at birth. *J. Small Anim. Pract*. **22**, 503-510.

Chapter 8

Some Problems of Parturition

It is customary to consider dystocia under the broad headings of maternal and fetal causes, and it is proposed to adhere to this division while enlarging the former to include behavioural factors.

MATERNAL CAUSES OF DYSTOCIA

Conformation of the dam

Certain types of conformation can produce maternal dystocia although this may not be due to small pelvic size as discussed below. The bulldog is one such example; the very large barrel-shaped chest with very deep costal arch is associated with a pronounced 'waist' and relatively small pelvic girdle although not necessarily a small birth canal. In heavily pregnant bitches the result is that the gravid uterus drops downwards and forwards in such a manner that the segment of uterus containing the presenting fetus is at a relatively acute angle to the pelvic inlet so that the fetus is not in an optimum position for easy engagement. Simple measures such as the application of a supportive sling to the abdomen or the elevation of the abdominal floor manually during straining sometimes result in delivery of one or two fetuses thus relieving the situation.

Abnormalities of the pelvis

Congenital factors

These include small size of the birth canal for the breed concerned, although this is very difficult to assess in any prenatal examination. Due to the enormous variation in the size of breeds there is no possibility of establishing criteria for pelvic dimensions hence pelvimetry is out of the question. The size of the birth canal is usually established by digital examination per rectum. The effectiveness of this method will depend to some extent upon the experience of the clinician with the breeds prevailing in a given practice area of both the potential dam as an adult and the size range of fetuses expected in the breeds concerned. This examination is often requested by owners and it is important that they should be apprised of the limitations of the method and the reasons for this state of affairs.

Although it would be expected that breeds in which show standards demand relatively small hindquarters, e.g. bulldog, Pekingese, would have pelvises of doubtful capacity, they are often found to have surprisingly roomy birth canals. Much more important is the effect of dorsoventral flattening of the skeleton seen in some breeds, especially when achondroplasia exists, when it may be found that the normal, somewhat pear-shaped, pelvic inlet with the vertical diameter exceeding the horizontal is modified so that vertical and horizontal diameters are equal or so that the latter exceeds the former. Bearing in mind that fetal head shape is, in cross-section, remarkably uniform, apart from the extreme brachycephalics, with the vertical dimensions being the greater, it is clear that flattened pelvic inlets create an obstruction to engagement unless the fetuses are unusually small for the size of the dam.

It is suggested that *developmental deformity* of the pelvis can follow some forms of juvenile osteodystrophy, but this is regarded as unlikely for two reasons: firstly, improved understanding of dietary needs has considerably lessened the incidence of the group of bone conditions classed as rickets; secondly, the osteodystrophy of kittens which may result in the so-called hour-glass pelvis does not appear to have an exact equivalent in the dog and certainly the author has never recognized this type of abnormality either ante- or postmortem.

Acquired causes

These are much more important, the outstanding one being fracture of the pelvis. It is well recognized that functional recovery even from very severe pelvic fractures is astonishingly good in the dog, but, whatever method of treatment has been adopted, a degree of deformity almost invariably persists and in most cases is sufficient to distort the birth canal to a significant degree.

The majority of pelvic fractures are sustained in road traffic accidents and it must be remembered that even well-controlled bitches do manage to escape during their oestrous cycle. It is therefore important in all bitches sustaining a fracture of the pelvis that a careful rectal examination should be made following recovery; in cases where there is no possibility of pregnancy existing this can be deferred until bone healing is complete, but if there is even a small chance that the bitch has been mated this should be done 3 or 4 weeks after the incident together with an attempted pregnancy diagnosis so that a course of action can be planned, thus avoiding the emergency of a severe obstructive dystocia. Alternatives are spaying as soon as is feasible or elective Caesarean section at term; the timing of Caesarean section in relation to labour will be discussed later (p. 94).

Abnormalities of the vulva

Failure of the vulva to enlarge normally during oestrus has been referred to earlier in relation to problems of mating, but if such bitches are successfully mated the infantile-type vulva occasionally persists during pregnancy and does not even relax at parturition. This causes problems usually confined to the birth of the first puppy in a primiparous bitch. The presenting fetus is clearly recognizable in the perineal vagina and the muzzle or hind feet may be visible at the vulva. Even vigorous straining fails to expel the fetus and the bitch is usually in considerable pain.

Digital dilatation and assisted delivery are adequate in the majority of cases but, in extreme cases, episiotomy may be required. Extraction of the first puppy nearly always dilates the tissues sufficiently to allow normal whelping to proceed.

Abnormalities of the vagina

These are decidedly uncommon causes of dystocia; the role of abnormal tissue bands in the vagina (Herr, 1978) and vaginal hyperplasia have been discussed earlier (pp. 25, 26). The presence of previously unsuspected vaginal tumours has been seen very occasionally as a cause of obstructive dystocia in older bitches; Caesarean section is usually required. On rare occasions trauma to the vagina from the use of forceps at a previous parturition can result in fibrosis sufficient to cause obstructive dystocia. Lesions outside the reproductive tract which have been seen to effect a maternal dystocia at the vaginal level include an unusually large urinary calculus and a massive lumbosacral exostosis.

Abnormalities of the uterus

Uterine inertia

Without doubt uterine inertia is the most serious cause of maternal dystocia and probably causes more anxiety to the small-animal clinician than any other single condition. The name is self-explanatory, implying failure of the uterine musculature to contract adequately at term. Aetiology is not precisely defined and may well be multi-factorial with mechanical, hormonal, physical and genetic components all playing a part.

The relative importance of the various factors can be argued in many ways. It is well known that single-fetus (and even twin-fetus) pregnancies often terminate in inertia, and it can be argued that this is due to mechanical factors with inadequate distension of the uterus not initiating labour or that it is due primarily to hormonal factors, possibly resulting from both maternal and fetal deficiencies. Equally so bitches which are exceptionally heavily pregnant occasionally show inertia presumed to be due to overstretching of the uterine muscle; certainly if the inertia is not total and one or two fetuses can be delivered with assistance whelping may proceed without problem.

Uncommon causes of under- or over-distension are deficiency of fetal fluids (*see* p. 84) or a dropsical condition of all fetal units, i.e. *hydrops allantois.*

Physical causes include poorness of condition of the dam, whether due to overweight and/or general flabbiness, or, less commonly, a debilitated condition. It is generally accepted by breeders that bitches should be in hard muscular condition to be ideal for breeding but unfortunately this may well be only lip service. Many dogs, whether show, breeding or pet stock, are these days in poor muscular condition, often due to inadequate exercise, and it can be very difficult to get management suitably modified under conditions of modern life.

Probably the most important factor is the hereditary one. The high incidence of uterine inertia in certain strains and families is sufficiently strong circumstantial evidence of its significance. It is only possible to incriminate heredity when a sufficient number of cases can be related to a particular strain, but once suspected there is a very clear ethical duty to stop breeding from affected lines and the veterinary surgeon must fearlessly advise accordingly. There can be no justification for perpetuating lines unable to give birth normally, from whatever cause.

When heredity is a factor inertia may occur in bitches in which none of the previous causes operate, i.e. they are in fit condition and pregnant with an average number of fetuses.

Primary inertia

Complete primary inertia

This exists when no observable signs of second-stage labour are shown. In many cases, especially in single-fetus pregnancies, there is absolutely no indication of parturition whatsoever; not infrequently it is assumed that the bitch is, after all, not pregnant. In this context routine 12-hourly temperature taking can be most helpful as the drop in rectal temperature may be the sole indication that parturition has come and gone.

In other cases there is evidence of first-stage labour but this is not progressive and signs become increasingly intermittent and more feeble and eventually disappear after an interval which may vary from 3 to 48 hours. Occasionally fetal fluids are discharged but no straining occurs. If the cervix can be reached digitally it is often found to be fully dilated but there is no reflex straining response to the exploring finger. These signs, in the absence of a positive diagnosis of pregnancy, may easily be mistaken by the owner for the behaviour of false pregnancy.

Complete primary inertia is an indication for Caesarean section which, if live puppies are to be obtained, must be performed early especially in breeds where fetal viability is low, e.g. Scottish terrier. If nothing is done possible sequelae include the following: the cervix remains closed, or recloses, with eventual mummification of the fetus(es) and resorption of fetal fluids; ossified remnants may be expelled many weeks after term; bacterial infection may supervene when signs typical of metritis are seen; if the cervix is open, dark greenish-black viscous discharge characteristic of placental separation is seen and is an indication for Caesarean hysterotomy or hysterectomy.

In all cases of complete primary inertia the prognosis for future whelpings must be extremely guarded.

Partial primary inertia

This is seen when there is some evidence of second-stage labour, usually as feeble, non-productive and purposeless straining, irregular in both periodicity and strength and no progress is made.

If it can be established that the cervix is fully dilated and if the number of fetuses is estimated to be small, only then is it justifiable to attempt medical treatment. Ecbolics, preferably oxytocin, are best given in small repeated doses by intravenous or intramuscular routes. The use of intravenous infusion technique is scarcely practicable in the restless, parturient bitch. Close supervision of the parturition by the veterinarian is necessary if administration of the ecbolic is to be intravenous, and this also is often not practicable. However, in selected cases and after careful clinical examination of the subject, it may be possible to rely upon the intelligent dog breeder to administer prearranged doses of ecbolic at prescribed intervals by the subcutaneous or intramuscular routes.

It is difficult to make precise dosage recommendations, but it should be remembered that physiological doses are very small and that the primed myometrium of parturition is highly sensitive to oxytocin hormones and can easily be overstimulated to an unproductive spasmic contraction. In cases of intravenous administration it is therefore safest to commence with extremely low dose levels bearing in mind, for example, that a single dose of 200 mμ oxytocin will induce parturition in the rabbit doe.

In the case of intramuscular or subcutaneous administration less precise attention to detail is necessary since the rate of uptake will be variable, but it is nevertheless prudent to restrict initial dosage administration to the lower end of the manufacturer's recommended range which is 2·0–10·0 i.u.

A combination of subcutaneous oxytocin, calcium borogluconate and stilboestrol (0·5-1·0 mg) is often preferred, the combination of sensitizing agents acting surprisingly rapidly but being less precisely controllable.

Results are variable from none to the delivery of one or two fetuses, which is satisfactory if the number is small, but there is always a risk of a fetus being left at the cranial end of a uterine horn necessitating eventual Caesarean section. In some cases medical treatment will bring a fetus to the pelvic inlet from where it may be possible to effect a forceps delivery.

Barrett (1949) reported on the action of intravenous calcium in inertia cases and it is possible that hypocalcaemia may uncommonly occur at or before parturition. Clinical signs are not always easy to detect in a bitch possibly already in first-stage labour. The author has seen one fully developed case in a 7-week pregnancy which it was impossible to follow through to parturition. If calcium deficiency is suspected it is justifiable to carry out a therapeutic/diagnostic test by administering a modest dose of calcium subcutaneously; a favourable response is an indication for continued calcium therapy.

The decision as to when to interfere in cases of primary inertia is one of the most anxious the clinician has to make and the criteria upon which to base this decision are few and difficult. Temperature drop followed by a dilated cervix is sufficient indication that parturition has failed and that surgery is required. Fetal viability as assessed by fetal heart rate is very valuable; slowing of the heart rate is a clear indication of fetal embarrassment and action must be taken. Unfortunately it can be extremely difficult to auscultate fetal hearts if it is a low-number pregnancy in a thick-walled abdomen and fetuses are thus not adjacent to the abdominal wall. If there is any doubt as to the existence of pregnancy in inertia cases radiography should be employed.

Secondary inertia

This is always partial since it is clear that second-stage labour is present as in most cases some fetuses have been delivered.

Although there may be some inherent tendency to inertia this is not always the case and it is often due to exhaustion of the uterine muscle in several circumstances, e.g. obstructive dystocia not dealt with sufficiently promptly, delivery of a largish litter containing some fetuses of relative oversize which have required more than average effort by the dam to achieve delivery of each.

Cases have been reported in which a long rest period induced by suitable narcotics has resulted in the return of muscle tone and whelping proceeding normally.

If the number of fetuses remaining in utero is small and there has been no evidence of oversize the use of ecbolics, possibly associated with the use of forceps, is entirely justified. There is a tendency to resort too easily to Caesarean section when a more conservative approach would be adequate, often as a result of owner pressure

Deficiency of fetal fluids

This is not common but has been seen on a number of occasions. Antenatal diagnosis is seldom made although in retrospect it is often clear that fetal outlines have been unusually easily palpable and that abdominal distension has been less than would be expected. In most cases no fetuses are delivered naturally but occasionally one puppy is born after much effort, covered in a tacky, blackish secretion. No fetal fluids are lost at any stage. At Caesarean section the placenta does not separate as expected and the fetus usually has to be 'peeled' out of its membranes. No suggestion is made as to aetiology. Two such cases were recorded by Joshua (1963).

Hydrops allantois

This is the converse of the above, with an excess of fluid being associated with each fetal unit.

The bitch is excessively distended in late pregnancy and may show cardiac and respiratory embarrassment from the gross intra-abdominal pressure. Caesarean section is usually required and such cases present an above-average anaesthetic risk; a fall in blood pressure due to the sudden decrease in abdominal content is also a complication. Whilst fetuses may be alive on delivery viability is usually poor.

Occasionally an affected bitch may, with assistance, be able to deliver one or two whelps per vaginam and the reduction in distension may allow natural progress, but the essential factor in dystocia due to this cause is probably severe overstretching of the uterine muscle making it incapable of normal parturient contraction.

Very unusual causes

Very unusual causes of dystocia include pregnancy in a herniated uterine horn which, for some reason, has not been dealt with at an earlier stage, and preparturient torsion of the uterus; the latter presents as an abdominal catastrophe in the heavily pregnant bitch and precise diagnosis may not be made until exploratory laparotomy is performed as an emergency measure.

The problem of the gravid inguinal metrocele presented close to term relates largely to the timing of the inevitable Caesarean delivery of the fetuses so placed. In the case presenting all fetuses inguinally, timing is of largely academic importance only, although with some regard to the desirability of approaching hysterotomy at the time most compatible with natural separation of the placenta. In the case presenting both inguinally and normally placed intra-abdominal fetuses, the relative merits of elective surgical removal of all fetuses or of the inguinal fetus alone must be taken into account.

There are on record cases of successful parturition of the normally placed fetuses of pregnancies following surgical removal, either at mid-pregnancy or immediately prepartum, of the inguinally placed fetus. However, in the majority of cases the decision is made to perform a total hysterotomy rather than face the risks attendant upon abdominal straining in a bitch recently subjected to surgical closure of the inguinal canal.

FETAL CAUSES OF DYSTOCIA

These are related to size, presentation (including position and posture) and fetal monstrosities.

Oversize

Oversize is defined as absolute or relative and the classical definitions are:
    Absolute — when the maternal birth canal is normal.
    Relative — when the maternal birth canal is small.

In view of the great disparity in size and shape of canine subjects referred to previously it is felt that these criteria cannot usefully be applied in the bitch. Hence it is preferable to regard *absolute oversize* as existing when the presenting part of the fetus cannot engage in the pelvic inlet, whether this be due to the large size of the fetus or to the smallness of the birth canal. *Relative oversize* is the term preferred when engagement is possible but progress of the fetus through the birth canal is difficult, i.e. greater than average effort is required for expulsion, or impossible unless assistance, whether digital, by forceps or surgical, is given.

The diagnosis of absolute oversize is based on the recognition of normal presentation, position and posture of the fetus accompanied by failure to engage even when straining is vigorous or instrument assistance is given. Absolute oversize, whether of the first or subsequent fetus, is an indication for Caesarean section, not removal piecemeal per vaginam.

Relative oversize is recognized by an obviously 'tight fit' after engagement and slow or absent progress. Although relative oversize can arise in any breed it is more likely to do so in breeds in which size has been standardized relatively recently (e.g. within the last 20 years) and in those varieties in which miniatuarization has been practised.

Treatment of dystocia due to relative oversize will depend upon several factors. If the first puppy is oversize it is undoubtedly justified to attempt assisted delivery per vaginam as (1) the remaining fetuses may be of normal size, and (2) the birth canal will be fully dilated for subsequent births. If, however, assessment suggests that the litter is a large one and the breed is one in which varying fetal size is to be expected, it is better to proceed to Caesarean section without delay.

The pros and cons of assisted delivery per vaginam versus prompt recourse to Caesarean section are infinitely arguable. Although with modern methods the latter is a very successful procedure and is undoubtedly quicker for all concerned, delivery by the natural route is preferable if this can be achieved without undue distress to the bitch, especially in primigravidae when the full development of maternal behaviour is so important. Assisted delivery per vaginam will entail prolonged and/or repeated attendance throughout the whelping to ensure prompt delivery of live puppies and to avoid unduly prolonged straining by the dam with the risk of secondary inertia supervening. (Details of a method of forceps assistance and of Caesarean section are given on pp. 92–100.)

Fetal monstrosities

These cause obstructive dystocia due to overall size, abnormal enlargement of a part or impossibility of normal presentation.

Anasarca

This causes a diffuse oedema of the whole fetus not only increasing its size but also causing a doughy consistence not conducive to easy delivery. Such monsters can occasionally be delivered per vaginam but Caesarean section is usually required.

Hydrocephalus

In severe cases a generalized enlargement of the head exists. This is commonly seen in the Pekingese as a cause of dystocia, but other breeds are also prone. If the affected fetus is in anterior presentation it may be possible to detect the fluid fluctuation digitally under the thin skull. Whilst surgery is usually required it is possible occasionally to puncture or crush the fetal head to allow escape of the fluid and then deliver by traction; this is not feasible in cases of posterior presentation.

Developmental anomalies of the abdominal wall similar to those found in *Schistosoma reflexa* occasionally occur, the fetus usually being in transverse presentation when the incomplete abdominal musculature and/or viscera can be recognized. Surgery is usually necessary.

Abnormalities of presentation, position and posture

When one considers the normal position of the fetus in utero (*see Fig.* 7) it is quite remarkable that the changes required for normal delivery take place so successfully, i.e. rotation of the fetus about its long axis to attain the dorsal position and the extension of the head, neck and limbs.

Presentation indicates the relation of the long axis of the fetus to that of the mother and can therefore be anterior, posterior or transverse. It must be re-emphasized that both anterior and posterior presentations are normal in the bitch.

Position indicates to which surface of the uterus the fetal vertebral column is related and can be dorsal, ventral, right or left lateral or oblique. Only the dorsal position is normal.

Posture refers to the disposition of the head and limbs of the fetus. Only the fully extended posture is normal, whether in anterior or posterior presentation.

Presentation

Whilst both anterior and posterior presentations are normal (*Figs.* 8 and 9), the former is more conducive to a rapid birth, especially of the first fetus. Engagement of the firm bony muzzle and skull in the pelvic inlet stimulates vigorous straining and fully dilates the birth canal for the body to follow through. In posterior presentation the more tapering and softer hind-quarters do not provide the same pressure on the cervical area nor is the canal so well dilated, hence some hold-up either at the pectoral girdle or the head is possible. In such cases the feet and part of the hindlegs are at or through the vulva, but repeated straining efforts result in little or no progress; the placenta has already separated so that assistance is required if there is no progress within, say, 20 minutes of the appearance of the hindlimbs. As immediate veterinary attendance is not always possible it may be necessary to instruct owners how to assist, emphasizing cleanliness

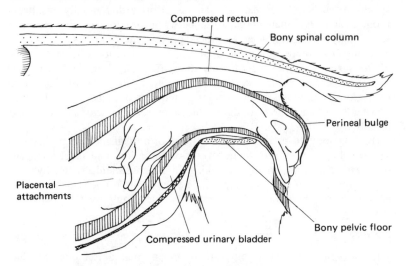

Fig. 8. Parturition with fetus in normal anterior presentation.

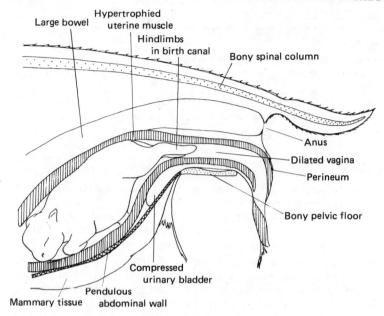

Fig. 9. Parturition: normal posterior presentation.

and gentleness. The slippery hind end of the puppy is best grasped, lightly but firmly, in a clean piece of towelling and traction is applied in a somewhat downward direction; traction should not be continuous but synchronized with the dam's straining efforts; this usually results in prompt delivery. Such cooperation between veterinarian and owner is surprisingly often possible and is much appreciated.

Transverse presentation inevitably causes obstructive dystocia; the body surface is more commonly presented and can be recognized by digital examination. Occasionally the fetus can be manipulated into dorsal or ventral presentation but this requires it to be repelled into a uterine horn and there is rarely adequate room. Caesarean section is usually required.

Radiography to establish the existence of a pregnancy often discloses a single fetus *apparently* in transverse presentation, and most clinicians will have had the experience of making this diagnosis and advising hysterotomy only to find the fetus perfectly normally disposed. The consolation is that a complete primary inertia probably existed anyway.

Position

The vast majority of whelps are in the normal dorsal position thus abnormalities are uncommon. The ventral position results from failure to

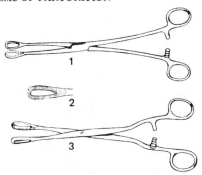

Fig. 10. Sponge-holding forceps.
Top – With box-joint, Foerster's forceps.
Bottom – With scissor joint, Rampley's forceps.
Inset – The elongated oval head of Rampley's forceps.

rotate upon the long axis (*see Fig.* 7, p. 66) and may affect only one or all members of a litter. Natural delivery is possible but is difficult and prolonged; surgery is often needed. Freak (1948) has described correction by the use of Rampley's sponge-holding forceps (*Fig.* 10).

Right and left lateral positions are rare. An oblique position is probably often attained during transit through the birth canal or may result from incomplete rotation and should not cause undue problems. Indeed delivery of a relatively oversized whelp can often be facilitated by rotating it through an angle of some 45° into an oblique position.

Posture

In this category fall the majority of abnormalities usually loosely described as malpresentations. For reasons of space it is not feasible to describe in detail all possible deviations from normal posture and only a few of the commoner types are described here. The interested reader is strongly recommended to refer to the classic articles by Freak (1948 and 1962) for extensive information on both this and the use of forceps.

Breast/head posture (*Fig.* 11)

The head is not extended upon the neck hence the muzzle of the fetus is below the pelvic brim and does not enter the pelvic inlet, the skull or nape being presented and recognizable digitally. Forelimbs may or may not be extended and in the birth canal.

Correction of this malposture is often possible using a combined forceps/digital technique.

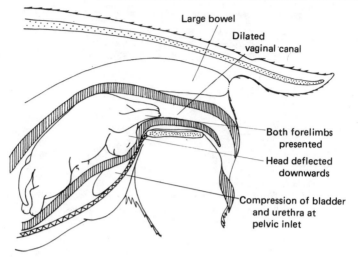

Fig. 11. Parturition. Fetal malpresentation with downward flexion of head and neck.

Lateral deviation of the head (Fig. 12)

This can also be recognized by digital examination and can often be corrected by manipulation provided the fetus can be repelled sufficiently.

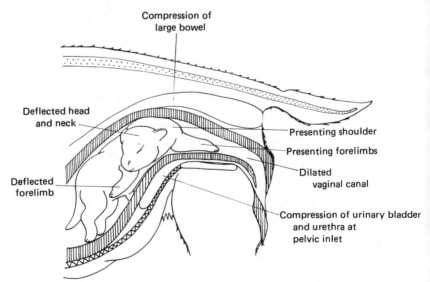

Fig. 12. Parturition. Fetal malpresentation with head and forelimb laterally deflected.

Forelimb(s) back

The head and neck have entered the birth canal but there is little or no progress due to the increased girth at the pectoral girdle caused by the unextended forelimb(s). This is one of the easiest malpostures to correct; using forceps on the upper jaw simply to prevent the fetus being repelled a finger is introduced and hooked behind the flexed shoulder so that the limb can be drawn forwards into the extended position. Delivery should then proceed spontaneously or with a degree of assisted traction.

Breech posture (Fig. 13)

This is a posterior presentation in which extension of the hindlimbs has not occurred and nearly always causes an obstructive dystocia. Vaginal examination discloses the tail and possibly the buttocks but no limbs. A combined forceps/finger technique usually corrects the posture fairly easily, the finger being introduced alongside the fetal buttocks and hooked round the anterior thigh muscles above the stifle; it is a simple matter to extend the hindlimbs and thus convert the malposture into a normal posterior presentation.

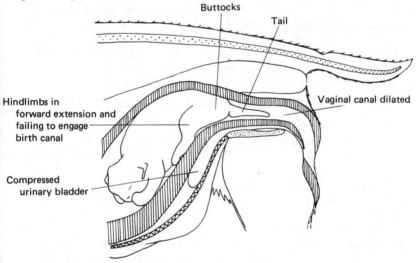

Fig. 13. Parturition. Puppy in breech presentation with tail and buttocks engaging birth canal.

PRINCIPLES OF TREATMENT OF THE DYSTOCIA CASE

Certain principles should be followed in dystocia cases. Care in the approach to whelping cases not only makes obstetrical work more rewarding but reduces the risk of litigious clients attempting to allege negligence.

1. Treatment should be based on a precise diagnosis of the cause of dystocia. This requires careful history taking and a careful and thorough examination. Probably the most difficult diagnostic problem is to decide if second-stage labour has commenced in inertia cases. This principle will be largely obviated in neglected cases.

2. The second principle is almost insultingly obvious, namely that all investigations should be clean. It is essential to insist on the provision of adequate facilities when dealing with whelping cases in the home; it is useful to specify these at the time of the initial call so that there need be no delay when the visit is made. New graduates are sometimes a little diffident in insisting upon such assistance.

3. Treatment should be embarked upon promptly (except in some cases of Caesarean section), bearing in mind that placental separation is commencing from 2 hours of second-stage labour onwards and that undue delay will jeopardize puppy survival.

4. The aim shall always be twofold; saving the life of the dam and delivering the maximum possible number of live undamaged whelps. With modern anaesthetic techniques for Caesarean section this is usually easily achieved.

5. The choice of method of treatment should cause minimal discomfort to the dam compatible with the desirability of retaining her active cooperation both in delivering whelps and in maternal care. Whilst Caesarean section meets the first requirement it does not fulfil the second.

6. Ecbolics should never be used in obstructive dystocia.

THE USE OF FORCEPS TO ASSIST DELIVERY

The types of forceps traditionally used for whelping cases have several disadvantages, two of which are that their size and mode of application greatly increase the dimensions of the fetus to be delivered and that they lack flexibility.

Rampley's sponge-holding forceps, referred to earlier, whilst not intended for veterinary use have several advantages when correctly used. They are made in two lengths (see Fig. 10). The grip is small, oval and ridged and the arms of the forceps on both sides of the joint are long, thus giving more flexibility. A box joint is preferable to a scissor joint as there is less likelihood of trapping vaginal mucosa. These instruments show a remarkable degree of variation in grip and flexibility despite their apparent uniformity. It is therefore wise to try several pairs before making a purchase; this is done by applying the grip to a finger-tip and closing the forceps so that the ratchet operates; the grip should be firm without causing much discomfort. A similar test can be carried out on a fold of skin of one's hand. It is often necessary to use more than one pair of forceps to effect delivery so at least two pairs should be purchased, preferably of different sizes.

The value of these forceps is twofold:

1. To obtain a grip on a presenting part of the fetus, e.g. the tail, hindlimbs or upper jaw, simply to prevent the fetus being repelled into the uterus while digital correction of a malposture is attempted, e.g. in a breech birth. When used in this way they should not involve much traction.

2. To provide assisted traction, e.g. in relative oversize via a hold on the upper jaw or, after extension of the hindlimbs of a breech presentation, to apply traction with the forceps applied to both hocks, *not* to the feet.

It is not proposed to detail the precise method for each size or postural problem but a few guidelines may be useful. The forceps should be applied only to the upper jaw when it is proposed to use traction; a finger in the fetal mouth will detect the ridges of the hard palate and so ensure correct application. It is all too easy to grip the lower jaw instead and whilst this grip may be utilized to assist repositioning of the head to facilitate engagement, the temptation to use it to apply traction should be resisted for two reasons: the direction of pull is not correct and damage to the mandible usually results – obviously the latter is immaterial if the fetus is already dead.

A grip on the tail should be used only to maintain position for other manipulation and never for traction. Whilst a grip on the feet is permissible if used similarly traction should not be attempted since the usual result is amputation. To apply traction to the hindlimbs the grip of the forceps should be applied around the hocks. Because this pattern of forceps is not space-occupying it is perfectly feasible to use three pairs at once, e.g. a positioning grip on the tail and a traction grip on each hock.

Given a degree of dexterity and the willingness to spend time on vaginal delivery a surprisingly high proportion of whelps can be delivered alive and undamaged by this method. If only one member of a litter is causing problems by virtue of oversize or malposture, attempted forceps delivery is very worthwhile; it is also valuable in providing assistance when slight relative oversize is a problem in several whelps and the bitch is having to exert undue effort for each birth, and in some cases of partial inertia.

CAESAREAN SECTION

This operation carries a very good prognosis both for bitch and puppies, especially for the latter due to modern methods of anaesthesia. Because of its ease and success there is a tendency to resort too readily to Caesarean section when other methods might suffice; nonetheless it is major surgery and as such should never be embarked upon lightly. A more detailed consideration of ethical problems follows later.

The routine surgical technique is well known, so details of technique are confined to a few selected aspects.

Indications

1. Pelvic abnormalities in the dam.
2. Vaginal obstructions, e.g. tumours or fibrous bands.
3. Uterine inertia; mainly primary but some secondary cases.
4. Absolute oversize.
5. Relative oversize if either the degree is great, the number of affected fetuses is likely to be large or there is evidence of inertia.
6. Malpresentations not amenable to correction.
7. Fetal monstrosities.
8. Single-fetus pregnancies with inertia.
9. Neglected dystocias.
10. Deficiency of fetal fluids.
11. Excess of fetal fluids, i.e. hydrops.

This list probably covers the more commonly occurring forms of dystocia in which hysterotomy is to be recommended.

Timing of operation

This is of importance and is to some extent controversial but must be related to the type of placentation in the bitch, i.e. individual, zonary or deciduate. Too early surgical interference can, and occasionally does, result in severe haemorrhage which may even be fatal. This consideration is most important in relation to elective Caesarean sections which, for ethical reasons, should be rare in veterinary practice. However, they are performed and it is essential that the operation should be timed, not to suit the convenience of owner or veterinarian, but in relation to the parturient state of the dam, i.e. in early second-stage or, if essential, in late first-stage labour. Only in cases of complete primary inertia is it justifiable to operate without evidence of the initiation of parturition; the problems of recognizing parturition in such cases have already been mentioned (p. 83).

When the second stage is in progress and it is clear that surgical interference is required there should be no delay. In cases coming to operation at an hour when adequate assistance may not easily be available the pros and cons of delay of a few hours must be conscientiously weighed against the possible effect of postponement on fetal viability, and these should preferably be discussed with the owner. A decision based on an honest assessment of the situation, even if it subsequently proves to have been mistaken, cannot be held to be negligent.

Given the existence of average skills and facilities, prognosis vis-à-vis timing can be assessed as follows:

Before 6 hours of second-stage labour: Excellent for the bitch and live pups with the possible exception of the first, in which placental separation is already occurring.

6 to 12 hours second-stage: Excellent for the bitch and most of the pups; very doubtful for the presenting fetus.

12 to 24 hours: Still excellent for the bitch but the first puppy will almost certainly be dead, except in some inertia cases.

24 to 36 hours: Fair to good for the bitch; poor for at least some of the litter.

36 hours onwards: These are mainly dystocias neglected due to ignorance on the part of the owner and the prognosis is now very guarded, at least for the whelps.

It is wise to give as accurate a prognosis as is reasonably possible prior to operation in order to avoid subsequent recriminations.

Anaesthesia for Caesarian section

Techniques can to a considerable extent be varied with each circumstance, bearing in mind both the over-riding objective of rendering the surgical subject immobile and pain-free and the ultimate objective of producing vigorous whelps to a dam rapidly able to provide mothering behaviour. To attain this, the drugs selected must be rapidly excreted or metabolized, must maintain good oxygenation of maternal and fetal tissues and cause minimum depression of both the cardiovascular system of the dam and the central nervous system of the fetus.

Drugs in general anaesthetic use are entirely suitable for these procedures, although they are often best used in combination rather than singly and with particular attention being paid to dose level in order to avoid excessive depression and problems associated with their metabolism and excretion.

Naturally, in some circumstances, the requirements of whelps can be disregarded and the anaesthetic technique aimed entirely at the wellbeing of the dam. In these cases routine premedication, induction and maintenance procedures may be adopted with, in many cases, additional treatment for the correction of peripheral circulatory failure. A suitable drug combination is atropine and phenothiazine derivatives as a premedicant, thiopentone or methohexitone as an induction agent and nitrous oxide/oxygen (50 : 50 mixture) with halothane as a maintenance inhalation agent. According to circumstance this regime may be supplemented by the administration of blood volume expanders and crystalloid solutions, the former preferably administered prior to the induction of anaesthesia.

In circumstances in which the wellbeing of whelps is of significance, the choice of agent for all stages of the anaesthetic procedure is debatable. On many occasions the exhausted and passive state of the bitch obviates the necessity for premedication, but when this is indicated it is probably safest to use a phenothiazine tranquillizer, such as acepromazine maleate, at a low dose level rather than narcotic agents with more powerfully depressant effects upon the neonate. Atropine may also be safely used although it can cause fetal tachycardia.

In many cases it is possible to eliminate the use of a depressant barbiturate induction agent by the substitution of inhalation induction using the main anaesthetic gas mixture administered by a face mask. When this is not possible, the rapidly metabolized methohexitone is probably preferable to thiopentone as an induction agent, although it is likely that when correctly used at minimal dose levels, the latter is less depressant of the neonate than imagined. However, whenever possible the use of barbiturates, even if only for induction, is best avoided.

For maintenance of anaesthesia it is customary to employ minimal levels of halothane in an oxygen/nitrous oxide vehicle, the latter being additionally useful for its analgesic qualities, but it is also possible to eliminate the use of halothane if muscle relaxants and controlled ventilation with oxygen/nitrous oxide are employed. Suxamethonium may be used at a dose level of 0·3 mg/kg intravenously to achieve relaxation of approximately 20 minutes' duration, which is adequate for the removal of whelps, after which, by the addition of halothane to the inspired mixture, a deeper plane of anaesthesia can be attained for the completion of surgery.

During inhalation anaesthesia a minimum of 30% oxygen must be maintained in the inspired mixture for the safety of the dam, and there are indications that higher percentages are preferable to ensure adequate fetal oxygenation. There is nothing to indicate that levels of halothane routinely administered in any way adversely affect uterine involution or predispose to postpartum uterine haemorrhage in the bitch.

In some circumstances neuroleptanaesthetic and regional anaesthetic techniques may be preferred, but by their reliance upon relatively limited numbers of agents on each occasion problems may be encountered with their use.

Associated with the narcotic effects of neuroleptanalgesics such as etorphine, fentanyl and thiambutene is the respiratory depressant effect of opioid drugs, both upon dam and neonates. Specific antagonists to these drugs may be successfully administered to fetuses following delivery, but most are themselves agonists in overdose and, since the requirements of each fetus are impossible to assess, may actually cause rather than reverse depression. The antagonist naloxone hydrochloride is devoid of this side-effect but has a short duration of action and may require to be administered repeatedly, an expensive and tiresome procedure. Despite the recorded depressant effect of thiambutene on neonates it was formerly routinely used as the narcotic of choice in association with regional block and was associated with the delivery of apparently undepressed whelps with a high survival rate. It is regarded by some as a very successful method.

Regional anaesthesia may be by local infiltration analgesia or epidural analgesia of suitably sedated subjects. This technique is acceptable in that the anaesthetic drugs employed cause minimal fetal depression, but it is less than ideal in that the requirement for sedation of the subject may necessitate the employment of unacceptably high dose levels of depressant sedative drugs. Regrettably, even the use of sufficient quantities of the relatively safe phenothiazine tranquillizers may occasion maternal circulatory problems and hypotension because of their α-adrenergic blocking properties.

Since the circumstances under which surgery is performed are immensely variable, it is impossible to prescribe a single preferred procedure although each surgeon/anaesthetist is inclined to favour familiar techniques. For fetal wellbeing it is clearly preferable to utilize minimum effective quantities of any drug selected, while for maternal wellbeing the greatest benefit probably accrues from additional attention to supportive treatments such as correction of peripheral circulatory failure and extravascular fluid deficits.

Site of abdominal incision

Both midline and flank incisions are in use. Many veterinarians favour the flank approach, using an oblique upward and backward or almost horizontal incision sited over the fetus nearest the pelvic inlet on the relevant side. The main reason for preferring the flank incision is the greatly decreased risk of wound breakdown; breakdown of midline and even paramedian incisions remains a hazard, even if only occasional, whereas this complication is exceedingly rare with the flank approach.

Advantages of flank incision

1. Rarity of wound breakdown.
2. Several layers of muscle at the incision site.
3. Greater vascularity of the tissues, therefore better and quicker healing.
4. No pressure of abdominal viscera on the incision line.
5. The incision is not sited between masses of active mammary tissue which in a nursing bitch is warmer and more moist than normal.
6. The muscular flank incision is more distensible than the more rigid midline fascial site, hence a much smaller incision will suffice.

Disadvantages of flank incision

1. More time is needed to enter and close the abdomen which may be considered unacceptable in an operation in which speed is usually required.
2. Some haemostasis is required although usually forceps pressure is adequate.
3. A large area of the flank is clipped which occasionally causes owners to complain, but owner preference cannot be allowed to outweigh surgical safety.

In most cases a single *uterine incision* is adequate, sited either in the uterine body or over the presenting fetus in the uterine horn. It is usually possible to manipulate other fetuses to the one incision. It is customary to incise the uterus over an extremity of the fetal trunk, avoiding the placental zone (*see Fig.* 7), but great care must be exercised as it is all too easy to damage the fetal skin which causes owners to complain out of all proportion to the seriousness of the damage.

It is vitally important that the uterus and vagina should be most carefully explored to ensure that every fetus has been removed. If this is criticized as being a statement of the obvious it can be categorically stated that cases in which fetuses have been left in utero following hysterotomy come before the Veterinary Defence Council.

The method of separating placental attachments as each fetus is propelled towards the incision is of some importance. A squeezing action applied cranial to the zone of attachment is preferable to the application of traction as it minimizes haemorrhage. To the same end, it is preferable in some circumstances, especially those of apparently firm placental attachment, to leave placentae in situ for subsequent spontaneous expulsion. When involution is adequate no other precaution regarding postoperative intra-uterine haemorrhage is necessary. In the event of delayed involution ecbolics may be employed, and it is in this precise circumstance that ergometrine was considered to be the drug of choice, having a more specific myometrial than cervical contractile action, in contrast to the ecbolics of pituitary derivation.

Handling and resuscitation of Caesarean whelps

It is essential to have adequate assistance available to deal with pups as they are extracted from the uterus which should be a pretty speedy procedure when most of the fetuses are viable; it is often possible at this stage to invoke the aid of dog-breeder owners who can be very valuable for obvious reasons. As each fetus is removed from the uterus it is customary for the surgeon rapidly to tear away the membranes from the fetal muzzle and then drop the puppy into suitable clean material held out by the assistant; a finger should be passed quickly through the mouth to remove any mucus and/or membrane and the puppy should be held with head downwards to ascertain whether any fluids have been aspirated during delivery. The umbilical cord should be separated 1-1½ in. from the fetal abdomen.

The next procedure is to instigate respiration which, in a vigorous whelp, will usually follow quickly as the pup is rubbed dry. If response is slow special attention should be paid to the parts of the pup to which the dam would normally devote her attention particularly, i.e. nose and muzzle, anus, vulva and/or prepuce and the umbilicus. Observation of normal whelpings demonstrates that respiration and crying result from such attentions by the dam and these should be utilized in resuscitation techniques. Provided the fetal heart rate is within normal limits resuscitation attempts should be continued for at least 30 minutes, but if the heart rate is slow prognosis is poor. Immersing the pup alternately in warm and cold water is claimed by some to be effective but the author has not found this to be of any avail when more conventional methods have failed.

After drying as thoroughly as possible pups should be put into a previously prepared box or basket in which a *warm* hot-water bottle covered by a piece of blanket has been placed; the whelps should then be lightly covered with suitable material. It is vital to bear in mind that the warmth essential to newborn pups should be provided by *contact* in order to simulate the heat generated by the dam's mammary area and the other whelps, rather than by a high ambient temperature of the much-loved and misused infra-red lamp suspended from above. There is no urgency to start artificial feeding.

Introducing Caesarean whelps to the dam

There is seldom any problem when the dam has reared a previous litter if her mothering behaviour was good. The pups can be put with her as soon as she clearly recognizes the sound of her crying offspring and has sufficient coordination not to damage them. This is usually within a very few hours with current anaesthetic methods. This regime has two advantages; first, the pups can quickly obtain colostrum from which they derive a high proportion of their maternal antibodies and, secondly, the act of suckling augments involution of the uterus.

The problem is slightly greater in the primigravida as there is no learned component of behaviour from previous experience and the normal stimuli provided by vaginal delivery are absent unless some whelps have been delivered naturally prior to operation. Most bitches have strong maternal instincts, and it is the firmly held view of many clinicians that continued breeding from bitches of poor mothering behaviour is unethical. If a bitch can be persuaded to lick her newly presented puppies full mothering behaviour quickly follows; the best method of ensuring that she will lick her pups —remembering that the alien smell of the operating table may mask the usual odour — is to smear them with a little of her own vaginal discharge which usually has the desired result. In the case of midline surgery, after removal of all surgical skin dressings from the mammary skin, the area may be massaged with a little milk expressed from the teats. In either case the bitch should be closely supervised until her willingness and ability to perform maternal duties are established.

Ethics

Whilst Caesarean hysterotomy is a reliable and successful operation which should be unhesitatingly performed as a life-saving procedure when no other method of delivery is practicable, its very success has led, especially in dog-breeding circles, to what can be regarded as a degree of abuse when assessed solely on ethical grounds. As indicated earlier the vaginal route has much to commend it in many circumstances, and should always be considered in dystocia cases. The most difficult problems arise in dealing with strains and breeds which have an unusually high incidence of dystocia, whether due to conformation or inertia. In instances where conformation is the factor many breeders are very ethical and select breeding stock for self-whelping ability; they should be strongly supported by the veterinary profession for so doing.

In other cases show-ring success is the over-riding consideration which may result in perpetuation of strains quite unable to whelp normally, thus resulting in a demand for elective Caesarean section. It is clearly essential that the operation must be performed if required in the first dystocia of a given individual but if, after careful assessment, it is obvious that there is a high risk of a repetition at the next parturition it is the duty of practitioners to advise strongly against further breeding and to refuse to carry out a series of elective Caesarean sections for a given breeder in such circumstances, even if it means the loss of a client. It is absolutely wrong deliberately to put a bitch in whelp when it is known that there is a risk of dystocia as, despite its success, hysterotomy is a major operation with all its attendant discomforts. Such major surgery can never be condoned for the pleasure and/or profit of the owner.

However, problems of advising owners arise in circumstances in which ethics are less involved, i.e. advice as to whether to breed again from a bitch which has had a Caesarean section. This advice must be based on a careful assessment of the factors causing the current dystocia and on what can only be called an educated guess about the future.

The following are some of the situations encountered:

1. Inertia believed to be due to a low number of whelps, i.e. one or two. Advise to try again ensuring maximum conception by multiple services; if the small number is repeated discard for breeding.

2. Oversize in several whelps. Breed once more to a different sire.

3. Malpresentation, position or posture. Unhesitatingly advise to breed again as these are often isolated incidents.

4. Complete primary inertia with no obvious contributory cause. The outlook is very guarded but it could not be regarded as unethical to try once more.

5. Partial and/or secondary inertia. This must be assessed on the facts of the individual case but it could seldom be regarded as unethical to try once more.

Owners are usually very appreciative of full and frank guidance following a discussion of the case, and it is fortunately only a small minority who will exert pressure in an unethical situation.

Caesarean hysterectomy

This is sometimes requested by owners in preference to hysterotomy, but is most usually indicated in cases of neglected dystocia in which there may be symptoms of secondary infection and toxaemia. Possibly because of this, the prognosis is less regularly favourable than for Caesarean hysterotomy and it would appear that the bitch tolerates Caesarean hysterectomy less well than does the cat in similar circumstances. Although this opinion is not universally accepted, it is often preferable to reserve Caesarean hysterectomy for such circumstances rather than to perform it electively.

REFERENCES

Barrett E. P. (1949) A preliminary note on the treatment of uterine inertia in the bitch. *Vet. Rec.* **61**, 783.

Dodman N. H. (1979) Anaesthesia for Caesarean section in the dog and cat: a review. *J. Small Anim. Pract.* **20**, 449.

Freak M. J. (1948) The whelping bitch. *Vet. Rec.* **60**, 295–301.

Freak M. J. (1962) I. Abnormal conditions associated with pregnancy and parturition in the bitch. *Vet. Rec.* **74**, 1323–1339.

Herr S. (1978) Persistent post cervical band as a cause of dystocia in a bitch. *Vet. Med. Small Anim. Clin.* **73**, 1533.

Joshua J. O. (1963) Absence of fetal fluids and dystocia in the bitch. *Vet. Rec.* **75**, 956.

Chapter 9

Problems of the Postpartum Period

UTERINE PROBLEMS

Retained placenta

Although ideally the completion of third-stage labour should be noted by owner observation, this is frequently impossible either because of random delivery of fetuses and membranes or because of secretive behaviour by the bitch.

During routine post-whelping examination of the bitch retained placental masses are sometimes palpable, but ability to do so is very dependent upon bitch size and the degree of uterine involution and in some cases it is impossible to distinguish thus between uterine subinvolution and placental or fetal retention. However, it is sometimes possible to aid the expulsion of retained masses by such transabdominal manipulation. It is also occasionally possible to use gentle traction on the fronds of membranous tissue detected by digital exploration of the vagina, and to combine this with a transabdominal manipulative effort. The use of ecbolic drugs alone may be counterproductive in long delayed post-whelping, but in the immediate postpartum phase may satisfactorily stimulate expulsion and uterine involution. In cases of doubt it may be worthwhile priming with oestrogens (1–2 mg stilboestrol subcutaneously) to secure cervical relaxation and heightened myometrial sensitivity.

Whereas failure of complete expulsion may contribute to delayed uterine involution and endometritis, there must be many cases undiagnosed in which there are no untoward sequelae, merely a protracted period of postpartum vaginal discharge.

Uterine eversion and prolapse

Though rarely diagnosed, this condition has been reported by Wynne

(1980) who has recognized two separate presentations within the immediate postpartum period. In the most obvious cases eversion of a single horn was seen to have occurred with protrusion through the vulval lips, but without any symptoms of distress except that in one case this event occurred before the completion of whelping and resulted in dystocia.

The second presentation was in small-breed bitches at the conclusion of satisfactory whelping of single-fetus pregnancies. Continuing symptoms of abdominal discomfort and straining, initially misdiagnosed as evidence of dystocia, were seen to be unrelated to the presence of a fetus. By careful abdominal palpation it was, however, possible to palpate within the uterine body a ridge of invaginated horn. In these cases the restraining effect of the non-gravid horn was judged to have prevented total prolapse.

Correction by abdominal and vaginal manipulation, although theoretically possible in the fresh case, is difficult to evaluate and it is probably more satisfactory to approach the uterus by laparotomy in order to use slight traction on the ovarian extremity of the horn.

In neglected cases hysterectomy may be indicated in the event of failure to retract the tumefied and damaged tissue.

Subinvolution

This is a very common sequel to whelping, often only involving a single uterine segment. It is seldom of much significance as regards the health of the dam, but poses problems in the diagnosis of a puppy remaining in utero or of retained placentae. It can be exceedingly difficult to differentiate a non-involuted segment of uterus from an undelivered fetus and if serious doubt persists the bitch should be X-rayed. It is also difficult to know whether or not membranes remain attached in the enlarged segment and it is usually only when involution finally takes place without the passage of any placental material that a decision can be made.

Postpartum haemorrhage

This is a relatively uncommon but very serious complication of the puerperium. Haemorrhage arises from several or even all sites of placental attachment and is associated with subinvolution, yet by no means all cases of subinvolution — and they are many — result in significant haemorrhage.

Recognition of the condition is often delayed for 3 to 4 days after parturition, masked initially by the usual postpartum discharge which is often quite copious yet not abnormal. By the third or fourth day it becomes obvious that the discharge is unusually haemorrhagic and in severe cases the bitch is already showing evidence of blood loss characterized by lethargy, pallid mucous membranes and a rapid, small pulse.

In medical treatment ergometrine has been the drug of choice — its withdrawal has already been referred to. However, refractory cases do not respond to medical methods and hysterectomy is then indicated. Needless to say major surgery involving a recently parturient bitch suffering from severe blood loss carries a most guarded prognosis but can be quite successful. The logical pre-operative preparation by transfusion of whole blood is, regrettably, usually not satisfactory as the transfused blood is lost via the placental zones and discharged vaginally literally as fast as it is put in. The value of prophylactic injections of vitamin K during the final weeks of pregnancy is difficult to assess. This treatment has been carried out with apparent success, but in an entirely uncontrolled manner, in bitches which were suspected, on the basis of previous whelping performance, of being high-risk cases.

Metritis

Inflammation of the uterus in the period following relatively un-complicated evacuation of its contents is limited to its endometrial surface. In cases involving gross uterine trauma, either occurring naturally or surgically inflicted, inflammation of the myometrium and serosal surfaces will occur and may also occur if the treatment of endometritis is neglected.

Endometritis

This presents most dramatically in an *acute form* especially following abortion, unhygienic whelping procedures and retention of fetal membranes. It is a serious febrile disease usually occurring within a few days of parturition and requiring immediate medical treatment.

The bitch is depressed and anorexic but with polydipsia, pyrexia and a copious, noticeably foul-smelling, mucopurulent vaginal discharge, usually of a dark colour. In some cases lactation diminishes and supplementary feeding of puppies is indicated.

Treatment with broad-spectrum antibiotics usually effects a rapid resolution and this may in some cases be further assisted by the administration of ecbolics to hasten uterine involution. As in all circumstances of their use, care must be taken to ensure adequate patency of the cervical canal to avoid the risk of uterine rupture; thus only very small doses of oxytocin should be initially administered. Uterine lavage, though reported to be useful, is difficult to carry out and potentially hazardous because of the friable nature of tissues in advanced cases.

Subacute endometritis

This may often pass undiagnosed, but is not infrequently encountered in bitches which have had a protracted, though not necessarily traumatic, parturition. In these cases the bitch may exhibit only vague symptoms of malaise, including occasionally indifferent mothering behaviour, but should respond rapidly to the administration of a course of antibiotic therapy.

Chronic endometritis

This is frequently symptomless but is probably responsible for infertility at subsequent mating (see pp. 20 and 159).

MAMMARY CONDITIONS

Mammary congestion

This occurs most commonly in bitches which are going to be heavy milk producers and are excellent mothers. Owners often mistake the condition for mastitis, and it has also been wrongly diagnosed as agalactia. It results from the sudden copious production of milk at first let-down and is seen mainly in the heaviest producing glands, the two most caudal pairs.

The signs are somewhat confusing and are initially mainly behavioural with the bitch in a state of conflict between her desire to nurse her litter and a desire to get away from them because of the discomfort caused by attempted suckling. She will tend to try and kick whelps away from the posterior glands and keep shifting her position; in a big litter some of the pups will not be able to feed. On examination the affected mammary glands are found to be diffusely firm and very warm but with no evidence of bacterial invasion; milk can be expressed from the teats only with some difficulty. Body temperature is average for the immediate postpartum period.

Treatment is solely by management although precautionary antibacterial therapy may be considered wise in order to obviate the risk of subsequent mastitis. The owner is recommended to apply warm fomentations (water only) to the affected glands and when they are really warm to massage and knead the tissue; the strongest whelps should then be held to the teats involved while the bitch is lightly restrained and reassured. A return to normality within 36 hours is usual.

Failure to recognize and deal with mammary congestion results either in drying off in the glands concerned, with consequent loss of lactation in the most highly producing area which can cause problems with a large litter, or in secondary bacterial invasion causing a frank mastitis.

Agalactia mastitis

This terminology refers to the virtually unresearched condition of failure of milk production or of milk let-down in the immediate postpartum period. That the condition arises through an upset sequence of endocrinological events is suggested by its relatively greater frequency following Caesarean section than following normal whelping.

No satisfactory treatment can be recommended, but because of the known stimulatory effects of oxytocin hormone upon mammary alveolar musculature, and by analogy with its use in other species, the administration of repeated doses of oxytocin has become routine. No dose recommendations can be made, but consideration must obviously be given to the 'side-effect' of myometrial stimulation by the hormone.

Initiation of lactation in late pregnancy or metoestrus is thought to be a result of the negative correlation between plasma prolactin and progesterone hormone levels, the former rising to support lactation and the latter declining to facilitate parturition. Interruption of this balance may therefore be envisaged, especially as a result of surgical intervention, while the continuing decline in plasma progesterone levels in the post-whelping or postsurgical phase may account for the eventual commencement of lactation after a period of delay. It is uncertain how great a part the suckling efforts of whelps may play in stimulating late onset lactation, or how great a part psychological factors may play in this phenomenon. On the assumption that all may be contributory, it is therefore advisable to manage the situation by placing the bitch in a calm and secure environment with encouragement to nurse whelps. In the event of their failure to stimulate lactation gentle manual stimulation of the mammary glands may be useful together with repeated injections of oxytocin hormone.

Septic mastitis

Inflammation of the mammary glands due to introduction of infection may occur during the suckling phase and so present problems of treatment. In the case of involvement of a single gland it should be possible to permit continued suckling of healthy glands by application of a protective cover to the affected part.

If possible, local therapy should be employed with the avoidance of systemic antibiotic therapy because of its likely effects, via the milk, on puppy intestinal flora. If systemic treatment is indicated care should be taken to avoid the usage of tetracycline antibiotics because of the risk to puppy dentition.

In the case of abscessation of single glands, the application of hot fomentation to encourage pointing and discharge is desirable and effective, together with local instillation of appropriate antibiotic ointments into the abscess cavity. Intramammary instillation via the intact teat-duct system is not feasible in the bitch.

In the rare situation of generalized septic mastitis it may be necessary to remove the whelps and to institute systemic antibiotic therapy in order to obviate the risk of serious systemic illness and of gangrene and sloughing of inadequately treated glands. In such a situation prolonged antibiotic therapy and some milking-out of glands is suggested to achieve total clearance of infection and to avoid chronicity and the likelihood of recurrence at subsequent lactation.

Puppy feeding

In the event of an overlarge litter, failure of lactation or loss of the dam, artificial feeding may be necessary. This is a time-consuming and exhausting exercise since during the first 3 weeks of life feeding at a minimum of 6 times daily is indicated. As discussed in Chapter 13 the proper conduct of the exercise also entails adoption of the system least likely to result in behavioural disturbances. To this end normal suckling behaviour should be encouraged, also adequate exercise of limbs and bodily contact with other whelps. Attention must also be paid to the stimulation of defaecation and urination, easily effected by cleansing of the anogenital area with damp cotton-wool pads. Wherever possible initial suckling of colostrum should be ensured. Several reliable brands of bitch's milk substitute are available but a fortified cow's milk substitute can be prepared. A useful recipe, based on that of Bjorck et al. (1957), comprises 800 ml. fresh cow's milk, 200 ml 12% cream, 1 egg yolk, 6 g sterilized bone flour, 4 g citric acid, 2000 i.u. vitamin A and 500 i.u. vitamin D. This mixture, prepared fresh daily, is fed at 38°C. By 2½ to 3 weeks of age self-feeding can usually be achieved and early weaning on to good-quality solids is recommended from 3 weeks of age onwards (Baines, 1981).

Puppy weight gains during the first 5 weeks of life are relatively enormous and a doubling of birth weight within 5–8 days has been reported. The weekly gains of a breed having birth weights of between 12 and 16 oz and an adult weight of about 60 lb have been recorded ranging from 1·5 to 2 lb per puppy per week between 2 and 5 weeks of age. At an average litter size of 6 puppies this indicates the bitch's requirement to provide nutriment capable of producing up to 12 lb of new body tissue per week during the suckling period.

METABOLIC PROBLEMS

During the puerperal phase there are considerable demands made of the metabolic processes of the bitch in satisfying, via her milk supply, the requirements of rapidly growing puppies. These demands, superimposed upon those already made during pregnancy, reach a maximum approximately 3 weeks postpartum in the immediate preweaning phase.

Throughout this period complexly interacting homeostatic mechanisms within the bitch are responsible for the maintenance of blood levels of minerals and carbohydrates adequate to satisfy the requirements of both lactation and of the bitch herself, even in the face of erratic or inadequate dietary intake. Although most bitches cope with these demands, even at the expense of their own body substance, it is logical that the stress be minimized by attention to dietary adequacy. In providing for these needs it is probably wisest to avoid extremes of vitamin and mineral supplementation which might be counterproductive, rather placing reliance upon a good quality and balanced food intake.

Temporary failure of homeostatic mechanisms can give rise to at least two syndromes which may coexist and which present confusingly similar symptoms.

Hypocalcaemia (puerperal tetany, lactation tetany, eclampsia)

Classic symptoms are of restlessness, nervousness or anxiety followed, within 8–12 hours, by ataxia, tetany and coma. Various related symptoms of panting, whining, irritability, muscle tremors, etc. may be seen according to the phase of the illness and to a lesser extent the temperament and situation of the animal. There is, in fact, a noted tendency for the condition to be seen in small, excitable breeds. In tetanic cases there may be marked pyrexia due to induced muscular activity and in some cases the complication of a secondary hypoglycaemia, although the degree of interaction of these conditions is debatable (Irvine, 1964).

Although symptoms present most commonly in the first 3 weeks post-partum, they may be encountered during late pregnancy or during parturition as an aetiological factor in uterine inertia (*see* p. 83). There is also a suggestion that a low-grade hypocalcaemia may sometimes be a complicating factor early in the postpartum phase, especially among nervous bitches apparently unable to settle to maternal duties. In this situation it may be uncertain which is cause and which is effect. The syndrome occurs because of a reduction in concentration of ionized calcium in extracellular fluid, and is not necessarily indicative of an absolute calcium deficiency. Symptoms relate to the effect which this has on cell membrane potentials, allowing the spontaneous discharge of nerve fibres to produce contraction of skeletal muscles. In the naturally occurring case, the cause of the reduced concentration of calcium in extracellular fluid is not well defined, but a temporary inadequacy of parathyroid function is suggested on the basis that in cattle the feeding during late pregnancy of high calcium diets has been noted to have a provocative effect on the development of hypocalcaemia during lactation, presumably by placing an excessive reliance upon intestinal rather than on skeletal sources of calcium. It is possible that the situation may also be exacerbated by the reduced availability of calcium because of its increased protein binding due to systemic alkalosis, as may conceivably arise due to persistent hyperventilation by a nervous bitch. However, the interplay of potentially responsible factors is uncertain.

Diagnosis

Because of the serious risk of death during tetanic spasm, either due to respiratory embarrassment or development of CNS damage secondary to the accompanying pyrexia, emergency treatment is required and the response to treatment is usually regarded as adequately diagnostic.

Laboratory aids to diagnosis are few, but in most tetanic cases serum concentration of calcium has been stated to be less than 7 mg/dl. Comparable levels of 4-6 mg/dl are measured in cases of hypoparathyroidism.

Treatment

This is by slow, intravenous infusion of calcium, usually as borogluconate. To minimize the risk of induced bradycardia or cardiac arrhythmias 10% solutions are usually used although the successful use of 50% solutions has been reported. The speed of administration is clearly relevant to this. In most circumstances 5-10 ml of 10% solution by slow, intravenous hypodermic injection is adequate for the relief of extreme symptoms and can be followed by depot intramuscular or subcutaneous injection of an equivalent volume.

In the event of a lack of response to calcium infusion, the concurrence of hypoglycaemia, possibly as a secondary consequence of muscular spasm, should be considered and in extreme cases anticonvulsants, like diazepam (Valium-Roche), or anaesthetics should be administered to control spasm. In these cases a natural resolution may occur subsequent to the enforced rest period and forced withdrawal of suckling whelps.

In the absence of medical treatment, the removal of puppies is a sensible course of action, although in most cases the bitch will, in any case, be too restless to permit suckling. Following successful treatment there may be relapse, though uncommonly, and with this in mind early weaning is to be recommended.

Some bitches or strains show a tendency to hypocalcaemia following all pregnancies, and although this might be a reflection of a management problem, it is debatable whether such animals should be retained in a breeding programme.

Because of the complexity of the homeostatic mechanism controlling calcium metabolism by the interplay of hormones from the parathyroid glands, i.e. calcitonin and cholecalciferol (vitamin D), it is impossible to make simple recommendations about dietary control of this syndrome. Moderation is preferred and the utilization of gross quantities of vitamin and mineral supplements is to be avoided. Regular feeding of a well-balanced, mixed diet with the addition of moderate quantities of sterilized bone flour should suffice throughout late pregnancy and the nursing period.

Hypoglycaemia

The possible role of hypoglycaemia in the exacerbation of uterine inertia has been mentioned already, and it has been suggested (Irvine, 1964) that, as in other species, a syndrome of hypoglycaemia with ketosis may arise in the bitch due to the stress of whelping and lactation. It is further suggested that because of the similarity of presenting signs, the syndrome may frequently be misdiagnosed as hypocalcaemia and indeed may respond to therapy with calcium gluconate. The rationale of such response is taken to be the partial utilization of gluconate to raise glucose status and the reduction of nervous and muscular excitement by the state of hypercalcaemia so induced, the latter acting to allow the return of full function of homeostatic mechanisms only temporarily failing to fulfil requirements. With normal blood glucose levels of 70-100 mg/100 ml, and highly efficient homeostatic mechanisms, the dog is rarely spontaneously placed in the situation where an uncompensated drop below 50 mg/100 ml provokes spasticity and convulsion. If the situation does occur, it may rapidly worsen because of the glucose-depleting effect of increased muscular activity.

It has been hypothesized that such muscular tremors as occur due to hypocalcaemia are the most likely cause of the hypoglycaemia sometimes seen to exist concurrently, and in the event of failure of standard calcium replacement therapy to achieve resolution of the syndrome, glucose replacement should be instituted as a further logical treatment. An intravenous dose of approximately 10 ml of 20% solution should achieve some effect.

With experience gained of both conditions occurring distinctly separately, it may be possible to differentiate clinically the sustained convulsions of hypoglycaemia and the hyperaesthesia and muscular tremors of hypocalcaemia. In cases of diagnostic uncertainty the administration of glucose rather than calcium replacement therapy might be preferred because of the lesser risk of cardiac toxicity so entailed. However, it is stressed that cases frequently present as genuine emergencies requiring immediate administration of the appropriate treatment in situations which do not permit laboratory confirmation of diagnosis by the measurement and comparison of blood levels of glucose and calcium. Because of the greater frequency of occurrence of the hypocalcaemic state, initial calcium replacement therapy is more usually undertaken.

REFERENCES

Baines F. M. (1981) Milk substitutes and the hand rearing of orphan puppies and kittens. *J. Small Anim. Pract.* **22**, 555–578.
Bjorck G., Olssen N. B. and Dyrendahl S. (1957) Artificiell uppfödning av hundvalpar. *Nord. Vet. Med.* **9**, 285.
Irvine C. H. G. (1964) Hypoglycaemia in the bitch. *N.Z. Vet. J.* **12**, 140–144.
Wynne M. (1980) Everted uterus in the bitch. *Vet. Pract.* **12**, 26-26.

FURTHER READING

Capen C. C. (1979) Hypercalcaemia hypocalcaemia. *Proc. Neth. Small Anim. Vet. Assoc.*, no. 11.

Chapter 10

Perinatal Puppy Losses

Investigation of the spectrum of factors contributing to perinatal and especially neonatal puppy losses is currently the subject of cooperative effort between the veterinary profession and the dog-breeding fraternity under the auspices of the Animal Health Trust. Such interest in this subject is a reflection of the fact that puppy losses, on relatively conservative estimates, are thought to run as high as 15 to 30%, although precise figures are unobtainable.

The problem is of complex aetiology and may be considered from several points of view; perinatal losses may, for example, be broadly subdivided into deaths occurring at or immediately prepartum and deaths occurring in the postpartum, neonatal phase. Alternatively, classification may be into two other major groups, regardless of their precise placement within the perinatal period; the first comprising all obvious and easily understandable causes of death, such as parturient accidents and major congenital lesions, the second group comprising all inapparent causes.

No system of classification is entirely satisfactory since it is apparent that many aetiological factors can exert effects across such artificially raised barriers. Currently the greatest effort is concentrated on investigation of the so-called 'fading puppy syndrome' with the 'fader' defined as a puppy apparently healthy at birth but failing to survive beyond approximately 14 days of age. This definition is, however, arbitrary and it might be considered more valuable in the long term to extend it to include the period between birth and attainment of relatively adult physiological and immunological status. Also, since it is already apparent that broadly similar aetiological factors may be responsible for both prenatal and neonatal mortality in some cases, it is proposed here to avoid the confusion of contrived classification and to discuss the subject of perinatal puppy losses under the three relatively simple headings of congenital defects, infections and management problems.

111

CONGENITAL DEFECTS

Congenital defects are those present at birth with their precise cause unspecified. In many circumstances they are of genetic origin, but teratogenic and other factors, including gross maternal malnutrition, may sometimes be responsible. Some congenital defects, particularly those involving the central nervous, cardiovascular and respiratory systems, may be immediately incompatible with life, resulting in death at parturition, while other, less gross ones might remain unnoticed until the subject is fully ambulatory. Often such defects may be first diagnosed during the routine clinical examination of puppies prior to vaccination, or as the result of obviously limited exercise tolerance. In this category are such conditions as thoracic flattening with varying degrees of sternal concavity and limited diaphragmatic function, and peritineopericardial herniation with similarly limited diaphragmatic function. Lesions of the nervous system may be central, including hydrocephalus of varying degrees, cerebellar dysfunction and peripheral neuromuscular transmission defects. Some cardiovascular anomalies such as patency of foraminae may be similarly diagnosed relatively late on, whilst others, like anomalous vascular ring developments, may come to light at any stage due to interference with oesophageal function.

More readily detected by the dog breeder, but surprisingly often missed even during routine postpartum veterinary inspection, are cleft palatine lesions with or without harelip. The coexistence of a harelip and palatine deficiency is usually obvious and its incompatibility with adequate buccal function apparent. Lesions of cleft palate alone may not be sufficiently severe to preclude suckling adequate for sustenance, but the presence of milky nasal reflux is almost invariably apparent. In such cases of partial clefting growth is stunted. In cases of complete clefting there is early neonatal death. There is clear evidence of the genetic origin of this lesion in many breeds and it is not unusual for whole litters to be affected.

Respiratory and suckling problems may also relate to various congenital lesions of the pharynx and oesophagus. Certainly, the extent of soft palatine and peripharyngeal stricture apparent as a cause of gross respiratory difficulty in young puppies of several breeds suggests the likelihood of this lesion as a cause of neonatal puppy loss in some cases. Oesophageal obstruction due to vascular ring anomalies, and oesophageal dysfunction either due to cricopharyngeal achalasia or oesophageal flaccidity are also causes of neonatal losses, either directly through malnutrition or indirectly due to secondary inhalation pneumonia.

The extent to which other anomalies of the gastro-enteric system such as portocaval vascular shunts are responsible for neonatal losses is unknown, but more obvious anomalies like imperforation of the anus, account for a certain number of losses.

Other congenital defects occur which are, of course, not immediately life-threatening, although in a serious breeding programme they may be indications for culling and some, such as gross umbilical or inguinal herniation, at the very least, may present severe management problems including the necessity for early surgical stabilization.

Teratology

The evaluation of teratogenic factors remains difficult in the bitch although there are well-authenticated reports of the teratogenic potential of some drugs and chemicals in the species. To what extent perinatal losses may thus be attributed is unclear, but with increasing awareness of the disease potential in the dog, it is now routinely included among those species reported upon in specialist literature, including a recent epidemiological survey of cleft palate (Mulvihill et al., 1980), and in standard texts (Heinonen et al., 1977) as well as in surveys of specific drug effects.

As a general principle it is probably best to avoid the administration of any drug during pregnancy and certainly, although precise information for the species may be lacking, it is advisable to avoid the usage of any agent, such as a corticosteroid, which is known to exert adverse teratological effects in other species.

Overlap between congenital and management categories of aetiological factors occurs in the syndrome of 'congenital malnutrition' which is described in several species, including the dog. In this syndrome, as a result of severe maternal malnutrition or due to lack of adequate maternal blood supply, possibly because of competition of placental space, a 'runting' phenomenon occurs with the animal physically miniature and disadvantaged at birth.

INFECTIONS

The extent to which perinatal puppy losses can be attributed to primary infections is debatable. It is certainly true that postmorten examination of many dead fetuses reveals evidence of viraemia or bacteraemia, and that some bacteria, in particular coliforms, are relatively often isolated. In many cases, however, positive confirmation of viral infection is not forthcoming, and the significance of the bacterial isolates is not established.

Viral infections

Several viral groups have been implicated in perinatal puppy disease, although symptomatology of infections has varied according to the route and time of infection and the degree of passively derived antibody protection existent in the individual. Even against a background of routine vaccinal protection of breeding stock, situations exist in which passive antibody protection is not acquired, possibly because of colostral deprivation, and in which nestling whelps are susceptible to infection by viruses normally considered to be well controlled.

The relationship between adenovirus type 1, the aetiological agent of infectious canine hepatitis, and puppy losses is far from clear and that of canine parvovirus infection awaits evaluation. Finally, the role of canine herpes virus remains somewhat equivocal, being positively confirmed as the aetiological agent on far fewer occasions than it is diagnosed.

Paramyxovirus infection

This is responsible for canine distemper and although its occurrence among nestlings with loss of whelps is no longer commonplace it can occur, although presenting symptoms may be atypical.

Adenovirus

This, like paramyxovirus, is included in trivalent vaccines for routine canine protection so that manifestations of the complete hepatic disease syndrome are now relatively uncommon. However, the virus is relatively robust and resistant to disinfectants so that contamination of premises can occur. In addition carrier states exist, and by its excretion in jetting urine the virus may become dispersed in airborne droplets and be thereby easily transmitted. Transmission by ectoparasites has also been hypothesized as has the possibility of transmission in utero by recently infected or carrier bitches, although this remains enigmatic. Lesions of vascular endothelium and areas of hepatic necrosis in dead or 'fading' neonates are not infrequently attributed to adenovirus infection.

Parvoviral infection

Parvoviral infection of neonates is apparently most likely to manifest itself as sudden death or as symptoms of cardiovascular incompetence relating to lesions of myocarditis, although symptoms of incompetence may not be apparent in nestlings, but are seen rather later at several months of age. Symptoms of enteritis attributable to small intestinal lesions are not common in nestlings but may be seen in recently weaned puppies. The effects of parvoviral infection during pregnancy are not well known, but fetal death and/or abortion may presumably be anticipated in severe cases. As yet there are no records of cerebellar damage of fetuses although feline parvoviral infection in utero is known to be responsible for lesions of cerebellar hypoplasia in kittens.

Herpes virus

Herpes virus infection and perinatal puppy losses are to some minds synonymous but, although widely disseminated throughout the dog population, it seems unlikely that this virus is as widely implicated in the perinatal disease syndrome as is sometimes suggested. However, although the incidence of this infection in practice may be unknown, its pathogenesis is understood as a result of experimental and field work. The existence of bitch carrier status has been established (Hashimoto et al., 1979), as has the possibility of placental necrosis and the potential for fetal infection with the resultant birth of dead or weak puppies. Neonatal disease as a result of postnatal infection results from the ingestion and especially the inhalation of virus and presents as an acute necrotizing rhinitis followed, within a couple of days, by necrosis of other organs due to acute vasculitis. Leakage of red cells from these damaged vessels accounts for a characteristically haemorrhagic picture at postmortem examination, especially of the kidneys, liver, intestines and lungs, but clinically the disease manifests itself as crying, weakness, anorexia, sometimes diarrhoea, later dyspnoea and death, and is thus indistinguishable from puppy death due to other causes. Because the virus replicates in vitro at a relatively low temperature, it is considered unable to do so in vivo in a subject with normal homeothermic mechanisms so that only the neonate during the first 2 weeks of life is able to support virus multiplication and viraemia. During this stage mortality is high although individual recoveries are recorded in affected litters. The avoidance of hypothermia in puppies at risk may be considered a sensible precaution, but is unlikely to reverse disease progress.

Viral shedding in urine and nasal secretions occurs for approximately 2 weeks post-infection and contamination will also result from the whelping of uterine carrier bitches. Viral life off the host is short and relatively close contact in the crowded kennel situation is ideal for transmission. Although clearly existent on a worldwide basis, herpes virus has been confirmed on relatively few occasions in the United Kingdom.

Bacterial infection

Similarly *Brucella canis* infection, although well established in the USA as a cause of infertility, and of perinatal puppy losses on a kennel basis, has yet to be identified in the United Kingdom. However, imported animals carrying antibodies to the disease have been detected and it seems likely that the infection itself will eventually be imported.

Presenting only a fairly limited problem confined to large kennel premises, the disease is usually manifest as a marked overall reduction in success rate, as measured by pup yield/bitch/year. To what extent reduced viability of puppies born is a factor remains debatable, some reports suggesting the few puppies born to have reasonably good prospects of survival. Control, complicated by prolonged carrier status and ease of transmission, both venereally and by contact, relies upon the exercise of an eradication or isolation treatment policy based on tube agglutination or rapid slide agglutination screening tests now commercially available. The latter are reliable in so far that false negatives do not occur, but they require more elaborate laboratory confirmation of supposed positives.

Other bacteria apparently implicated in neonatal losses include *staphylococci* and *pseudomonas* species, both occasionally related to symptoms of enteritis and septicaemia, and, more commonly, *Escherichia coli* and *beta haemolytic streptococci* related to remarkably similar symptoms. Clinical differentiation of these cases is virtually impossible, and as a result misdiagnosis is common. In particular, like herpes virus infection, beta haemolytic streptococcal infection is frequently erroneously claimed to be responsible for perinatal losses, although there is no doubt of its aetiological significance on many occasions.

Other infections

Individual cases have been reported in which fungal isolates from the placentae of dead or ill-thriving puppies have been suggestively implicated as aetiological.

Roundworm (Toxocara canis)

Roundworm infestation of puppies is common in spite of routine deworming of bitches, and in some cases the weight of the intestinal burden is detrimental to healthy puppy growth. Occasionally the problem is more severe, the visceral migration of larvae causing gross, sometimes fatal, pulmonary damage.

Ectoparasites

The rapid infestation of neonates with ectoparasites can also occur, and this, in fact, is the stage of transference of demodectic mange mites. Neonatal death due to ectoparasitism is not, however, usual, although newly weaned puppies are not infrequently presented exhibiting well-established lesions of sarcoptic mange mite infestation and sometimes severely debilitated by louse and flea burdens.

MANAGEMENT PROBLEMS

Perinatal mortality may be associated with mismanagement of the bitch during pregnancy, mismanagement of whelping, mismanagement of the nursing bitch, the accommodation of the litter, etc. In many cases this final aspect is particularly relevant to failure by even easy whelping bitches to show good mothering behaviour.

The pregnant and parturient bitch

Mismanagement might in some cases pre-date pregnancy, e.g. failure to rear the bitch adequately and attend to her requirements for vaccination, deworming, etc. Mismanagement of pregnancy includes failure to maintain a state of fitness and to provide for dietary requirements. Mismanagement of whelping includes failure to provide an environment suitable for undisturbed whelping, undue manual interference at whelping and failure to detect the necessity for veterinary intervention in cases of dystocia, uterine inertia, etc. Also, in some breeds, failure to assist the bitch in severance of the umbilical cord and removal of fetal membranes from the head and airways constitutes mismanagement of whelping. Even in correctly managed whelping, however, it is not unusual for apparently perfectly formed puppies to be delivered dead and in these circumstances the precise cause of death usually remains obscure. Premature placental separation is often hypothesized as likely, but against this are the numerous occurrences of delivery of live puppies in unfavourable circumstances in which placental detachment of relatively long standing may be assumed. Certainly, relatively long periods of anoxia have been stated to be of little consequence to the neonate.

Ideal standards of management are sometimes difficult to adhere to, especially for the novice owner, but failure in this area should be obvious following veterinary assessment of the situation and can usually be rectified on future occasions by the application of common-sense principles as advocated elsewhere in this book. Mismanagement of the nursing bitch can also take several forms. Most obviously, failure to obtain veterinary treatment of hypocalcaemia, endometritis, mastitis, etc. may have fatal consequences for both bitch and whelps, and failure to deal with mammary discomfort may lead to reduced nursing.

At a more basic level, failure to meet the dietary requirements of the bitch may have deleterious effects on whelps, though this is unusual, rather giving rise to very marked depletion of maternal bodily reserves. Failure to take account of psychological disturbance to the bitch can have far-reaching consequences. This may manifest itself, as stated elsewhere, as the absence of normal mothering behaviour, overmothering with excessive grooming, aggression towards whelps and even cannibalism. Whereas these conditions are sometimes responsive to ataractic drug therapy, there is often a more significant response to improved management techniques, especially re-siting of the nest box in a position of greater security. Mothering problems may also, however, relate to the overzealous provision of extraneous heat. In these circumstances excessive heat dissuades the bitch from remaining with the whelps in a normal fashion.

The provision of ideal environmental conditions for whelping, nursing and rearing maximum numbers of puppies can be a problem. On the one hand, single pet bitches which are rarely faced with the hazards associated with 'dog-sick' kennel premises not infrequently refuse to utilize selected quarters, preferring less suitable locations and thus creating management problems. In kennels problems are far more likely to be those of environmental contamination, with a whelping unit in continuous use by a succession of bitches. Also in some circumstances problems can arise due to the minimal provision of secluded security and the minimum of bedding material and comfort so that chilling of puppies can occur.

Thermoregulation

The aspects of contamination relevant to infection and death of neonates have already been dealt with, but it is probably true to say that, these apart, hypothermia is the other major aetiological factor in neonatal disease and death. Crighton (1968) described the limitations of thermoregulatory mechanisms in young puppies which make them so dependent upon external heat sources. It seems probable that a 'zone of chemical regulation' so essential in adults for the combat of chilling by increased physiological production of heat (i.e. by shivering) is absent at birth. It is likely that to compensate for this lack, the puppy reflexly moves towards shelter and an external heat source when exposed to chilling. Experimental evaluation suggests a progressive change towards adult homeothermic capability by approximately 3 weeks of age.

Under conditions of natural whelping, a puppy ignored by its dam and repeatedly wetted by fetal fluids may become markedly hypothermic for a period of hours unless the ambient temperature is at least 80°F. In practice so high a temperature is unnecessary as long as the bitch shows good mothering behaviour, and indeed may be counterproductive in dissuading her from doing so. Close puppy contact with the mammae provides adequate extraneous heat, the glands being warm to the touch at a surface temperature only a few degrees lower than the bitch's own deep rectal temperature.

Because of bitch restlessness during whelping, puppy temperature in fact tends to oscillate between hypothermia and normothermia during this early phase. In the long term, however, in spite of confusing contradictory reports on the precise physiological interaction of hypothermia, anoxia and hepatic metabolism, it is clear that sustained hypothermia is detrimental to puppy metabolism as assessed by weight gain, cardiac function, etc. A healthy puppy is relaxed and laterally recumbent with a warm, sleek coat, bright-red mucosae and good muscle tone. It is capable of strong movement and suckling. Chilled puppies become noisy, and initially overactive, with an increased respiration rate from about 20 to 40/min and decreased rectal temperature from approximately 96°F to as low as 70°F. Although active, chilled puppies suck less well. Interestingly, this tell-tale sequence is not apparent in the immediate postpartum phase, but only in puppies that have initially warmed up adequately.

This state remains reversible with the supply of outside heat, but as temperature falls to between 70 and 50°F the reflexes are lost and there is increasing torpor with 'bronzing' of mucosae. It is suggested that previously healthy puppies may be retrieved from deep hypothermia of relatively long duration if rewarmed only very gradually.

To what extent hypothermia worsens the effects of intercurrent infections remains debatable. To obviate the hazard of this form of stress within the first 3 weeks of life, it is essential to encourage good mothering activities by the provision of comfortable nesting quarters and to avoid extreme fluctuations of ambient temperatures which tend to fall particularly low at night. If open whelping boxes are used, a night-time temperature of 70°F minimum is advocated during the first week.

Artificial heat is best provided by a source beneath the whelps to obviate the risk of cooling convection currents caused by overhead sources which may also reduce mothering. A moderate heat of this nature is provided by veterinary heating pads now widely available.

In spite of this accumulated evidence, however, many litters are successfully reared in normal domestic situations without the provision of supplementary sources of heating.

The need for external heat sources may also be obviated by the use of lidded and insulated whelping boxes with good heat retaining properties. In the event of use of artificial rearing systems, it is advisable to maintain ambient temperatures at 85°F for the first week, gradually reducing thereafter to 70-75°F by the fourth week. Puppies reared thus, particularly if deprived of colostrum, should also be retained in isolation and vaccinated at an early age, probably at about 6 weeks.

In *summary*, it would appear that the highest success rate should be anticipated from the well-maintained household bitch as long as she is free from psychological disturbance and is sensibly confined in a comfortable environment free from extreme temperature variation. To take this a stage further, a lower incidence of congenital problems is to be anticipated if the litter is the product of a total outcross mating. Since in some breeds derivation from a limited genetic pool makes this impossible, it has to be accepted that congenital defect is an ever-present possibility to be controlled by sensible culling.

Because of the complexity of the problem as outlined, it is difficult to advocate a single ideal approach to the investigation of a 'fading puppy' situation, but for practical purposes that outlined in Table 3 might be considered useful. Table 4 contains normal physiological values for neonate puppies.

Clearly, the performance of some of these requirements exceeds the facilities of the average general practice and in this event referral consultation is indicated. As has already been mentioned, such investigation currently forms the basis of a project at the Animal Health Trust's Small Animal Centre at Newmarket from whence helpful assistance may be anticipated.

Table 3. An approach to the investigation of a 'fading puppy' situation

1. Obtain a detailed case history of the incident in question.
2. Obtain a detailed breeding history of the bitch, and of all other kennel bitches; also a history of their vaccinal status and of any kennel disease problems.
3. Perform a thorough clinical examination of the bitch including routine blood biochemistry and bacteriological swabbing of the reproductive tract and tonsils. Assess immunological status when possible.
4. Visit the premises to obtain a personal assessment of conditions prevailing.
5. In the event of availability of fresh placentae or neonates perform appropriate histopathological and microbiological examinations. In the event of their non-availability, supply preservative so that at subsequent parturition placental tissues can be suitably preserved. Advise on the necessity of delivery of fresh, not deep-frozen, puppy carcases for examination.
6. Perform detailed postmortem examination of puppies and obtain microbiological swabbings of heart blood and contents of body cavities, as well as detailed histo-pathological examination of major organ tissues.

Table 4. Normal physiological values for neonates

Body temperature	Rectal 96°F at 1 day progressing to approx. 100°F at 7 days.
Respiration rate	20/min at 1 day (15–35/min).
Heart rate	200$^+$/min at 1 day.
Shivering reflex	6–8 days.
Muscle tone	Upright with tone and postural reflexes at 3 weeks. Rapid, coordinated movement at 4 weeks.
Eyes open	12–15 days (invariably blind if open at birth).
Focusing	At 21–28 days.
Ears open	13–17 days.

REFERENCES

Crighton G. W. (1968) Thermal regulation of the new-born dog. *J. Small Anim. Pract.* **9,** 463.

Hashimoto A., Hirai K., Okada K. et al. (1979) Intrauterine infection of Canine Herpes Virus. *Am. J. Vet. Res.* **40,** 1236.

Heinonen O. P., Sloan D. and Shapiro S. (1977) *Birth Defects and Drugs in Pregnancy.* Publishing Sciences Group Inc., Littleton, Mass.

Mulvihill J. J., Mulvihill C. G. and Priester W. A. (1980) Cleft palate in domestic animals: epidemiological features. *Teratology* **21,** 109–112.

FURTHER READING

Fox M. W. (1966) *Canine Pediatrics.* Charles C. Thomas, Illinois.

Chapter 11

The Male

In the dog, the male genital organs comprise a scrotum, two testes each with associated epididymis, ductus (vas) deferens and spermatic cord, a single accessory gland — the prostate, an urethra, penis and prepuce.

SCROTUM

Scrotal anatomy and physiology

The membranous scrotal pouch is divided into two cavities by a median septum comprising all layers except skin. It lies relatively far back between the thighs and, although protected by them, is visible and accessible from the perineal aspect. Each scrotal chamber contains the ipsilateral testicle (testis), epididymis, distal vas deferens and associated blood vessels. Beneath the scrotal skin there is a sheet of poorly developed smooth muscle tissue, the dartos, which by its contraction occasionally applies the scrotal covering more closely to its testicular contents. Dorso-medially within each cavity, at the point of attachment and reflection of its serous lining surface, is inserted a muscle, the cremaster, originating from the caudal border of the ipsilateral, internal abdominal oblique muscle, and running down within the spermatic cord. By their contraction the cremasters elevate the scrotum and its contents into closer contact with the abdominal wall.

The glandular, secretory nature of the thin, hairless, scrotal skin, together with this contractile capacity of the dartos and cremaster muscles, constitutes a mechanism for temperature regulation of the testes.

The serous lining of each scrotal cavity is an evagination of the peritoneum. The peritoneal and scrotal cavities retain connection through the inguinal ring and canal. A further invagination of this serosa envelops the testis, epididymis, vas deferens, associated vasculature and cremaster muscle, these last three constituting the spermatic cord.

The scrotal ligament, a vestige of embryonic gubernaculum, runs from the scrotal wall to the caudal extremity of the testis between the caudal reflections of the serosal tunic, though outside the serosal cavity itself. Together with the spermatic cord at the opposite pole, this ligament and the reflected scrosal tunics provide stability for the testis within the scrotal cavity. In fact, the potential serous cavity within each scrotal chamber exists only as capillary space between the serous surfaces except in cases of pathology, in particular herniation of abdominal contents through the inguinal canal.

Scrotal pathology

The scrotum is very susceptible to various forms of trauma, including dog bites, and such lesions are dealt with on routine lines. The scrotal skin is subject to neoplasia, often malignant. Both carcinomas and melanomas occur and whilst most cutaneous melanomas of the dog are relatively benign this is not always true of the scrotal site. The main clinical sign is intermittent but recurrent haemorrhage from the scrotum, and this is sometimes refractory to routine haemostasis; the underlying lesion has often not been recognized previously, especially in dogs with pigmented skin. Treatment is surgical and should be fairly radical, by excision of the affected area of scrotal skin ensuring that section is made in healthy tissue. Unilateral castration is often required and even total amputation of the scrotum with bilateral castration may be necessary; this is of little consequence in most patients since it is usually older age groups which are affected.

TESTES

Anatomy

The paired testes are oval in shape and slightly thicker dorsoventrally than from side to side, in normal position being situated obliquely with the long axis dorsocaudally. Because of their situation in the limited space between the thighs, they are usually placed one behind the other rather than side by side, the left testicle more frequently being caudal, but they may be symmetrically placed if low hung in conditions of total relaxation of the cremaster and dartos muscles.

The epididymis is attached to the dorsolateral testicular surface, its head situated cranially and its tail and spermatic cord situated caudally. Deep to the serous membranous surface of the testis is a dense fibrous capsule, the tunica albuginea, which is highly vascularized in its deepest layer. At the point of cranial epididymal attachment this fibrous tunic joins a testicular mediastinum of connective tissue lamellae supporting wedges of active seminiferous tubular tissue. These non-connective tissue elements comprise the sperm-producing tubular lining cells, their metabolic support (Sertoli) cells and interstitial (Leydig) cells which produce testosterone hormone. Aggregation of collecting tubules constitutes the rete testis within the mediastinum, from which tubular secretory products pass on into the epididymis with the assistance of circular smooth muscle contractile elements. Sympathetic nerve and arterial blood supply and venous and lymphatic drainage are all via the testicular mediastinum, these elements being carried within the spermatic cord at which level the testicular drainage vein forms an extensive pampiniform plexus around the others.

Physiological control of the testes

Although testicular function is fundamentally under pituitary control by the secretion of gonadotrophins LH and FSH, the intricacies of their interrelationships remain enigmatic. LH is known to stimulate Leydig cells to secrete androgens, while FSH stimulates growth and increased diameter of seminiferous tubules. In the absence of LH spermatogenesis does not occur, an effect presumably related to Leydig cell release of androgens, which are also necessary for the progress of maturation of spermatozoa within the epididymes.

The extent of effective feedback on hypothalamic function is equivocal since unphysiologically high dose levels of androgens seem necessary to achieve the effect by systemic administration. This is further complicated by the fact that whereas the inhibitory dose level suppresses LH release and Leydig cell function, with consequent aspermogenesis, a higher dose level, while remaining inhibitory of LH release, will itself substitute for the diminished Leydig cell function and so stimulate further spermatogenesis. Because of the relative grossness of these testosterone-dependent effects, it is therefore postulated that an as yet undiscovered inhibitory hormone of testicular origin may be responsible for feedback control. In several species, most noticeably cattle, it has been established that olfactory and visual stimuli may be responsible for the immediate release of LH and a precopulatory upsurge in blood levels of testosterone.

The role of prostaglandins in the male remains enigmatic, particularly in the dog which lacks the accessory sexual organs with which the hormones have been tentatively associated in other species. The high concentration of these hormones in human seminal fluid and their supposed prostatic site of origin resulted in the nomenclature of the series, but it remains debatable to what extent they might participate in ejaculatory processes, evacuation of accessory glands and assistance of seminal progress within the female.

Testicular descent

There is much misunderstanding amongst laymen regarding the age of descent of testicles and cryptorchidism, and it is important that the profession should be precise in their guidance on these matters.

The author has dissected a goodly number of male puppies between birth and 14 days of age and agrees with the findings of Arthur (1956) as quoted by Ashdown (1963). At birth the testes are still intra-abdominal but are usually near the internal inguinal ring; from 2 to 10 days of age they are descending through the inguinal ring and between 10 and 14 days have reached the scrotal area, bearing in mind that there is as yet no development of the scrotum. At this stage the testes can often be palpated in that region as discrete bodies some 0·25–0·5 cm in diameter. From 4 weeks of age onwards well-reared puppies lay down considerable fat deposits in the scrotal area which, in many cases, prevents precise recognition of the gonads, hence the common claim of breeders that they have not yet descended. Ability to palpate testes between 4 and 16 weeks of age is extremely variable as is the age at which pubertal enlargement starts. Some puppies of 4 months already have sizeable testes in a partially sacculated scrotum whereas other pups at 8–9 months have relatively undeveloped testes and a poorly differentiated scrotum. In these age groups there can be much difficulty in establishing entirety or otherwise in puppies intended for export although from 6 months onwards most dogs will have two well-developed testes fully descended into the scrotum. Veterinary opinion is often sought at shows as to the entirety of puppy exhibits and the following criteria are suggested as guidelines.

Terminology

Breeders should be encouraged to use the terms 'uni-' or 'bilateral cryptorchid' rather than the inaccurate 'monorchid'. Gonads in both sexes are paired organs and congenital absence of one gonad is exceedingly rare and in any case can only be diagnosed following a detailed postmortem examination.

Position of testes

Puppies cannot be exhibited before 6 months of age in Great Britain hence exhibits should have both testicles descended into the scrotum, with one proviso: the inguinal tissues apparently remain somewhat slack until approximately 10 months of age so that a testicle can be withdrawn or repelled into the groin hence a dog at first sight may seem to be a unilateral cryptorchid. Observation suggests that the left testicle is most commonly affected. Careful examination discloses the testicle in the inguinal area lateral to the penis and, if the dog is normal, it can be drawn into the scrotum into which it should drop easily. If the testicle tends to remain poised at the entrance to the scrotum and needs a good deal of traction to complete scrotal positioning, it is suggested that this should be regarded as being short-corded and interpreted as a minor degree of cryptorchidism.

Size of testes

As the time of puberty is variable it is difficult to be dogmatic about the age at which testicles should be expected to have attained adult dimensions. It is not uncommon to find 5-month-old puppies with apparently fully developed testes and this is confirmed by records of matings at that age being fertile. Equally dogs of 8–9 months may have small testes and it is suggested that with the exception of known late maturing breeds this should be considered as of doubtful normality. Not only is there a variation in the degree of testicular maturity between breeds but also between individuals in a given breed. A marked disparity between the size of the testicles should be regarded as abnormal.

Testicular pathology

Cryptorchidism

Both uni- and bilateral cryptorchidism regularly occur in the dog and the incidence is noticeably higher in some breeds suggesting a genetic component in its aetiology. There is still much controversy on this aspect and any attempt to breed out the condition is complicated by the probability that female siblings of a cryptorchid dog may carry a genetic factor. Nonetheless it is most strongly urged that abnormal males should not be used for breeding.

It is difficult to understand why criteria that are rigorously applied to and accepted for males of other species of livestock should not be equally applied to the dog and it is regrettable that under the rules of the English Kennel Club an affected subject may be exhibited and used for breeding.

Many breeders will claim that as a unilateral cryptorchid is usually fertile he cannot be regarded as abnormal; they cannot appreciate that fertility is not an important criterion. Most bilateral cryptorchids are, for obvious reasons, sterile.

The markedly higher incidence of testicular tumours in undescended testes, whether these be retained in the intra-abdominal or inguinal sites, is now well documented. For this reason it is suggested that the retained testicle should be removed by elective castration before the dog is 6 years of age in average breeds as this will, in the vast majority of cases, anticipate neoplastic change. In dogs with a shorter average life expectancy, e.g. bull breeds, removal of the abnormal testis should be earlier, e.g. before 4 years; the boxer, with an acknowledged high incidence of cryptorchidism, is included in this category. There is no reason why the normally descended testis in unilateral cases should not be left in situ so that any disadvantages of a neuter state need not arise. Quite apart from any consideration of soundness in conformation the acknowledged significantly increased incidence of neoplasia in undescended testicles is sufficient ground to make every effort to reduce cryptorchidism in the dog population.

Testicular tumours

Testicular neoplasia is quite common in the dog, this species probably having the highest incidence of any domesticated mammal, largely due to the fact that a high proportion of most other species are castrated early in life. There are three commonly recognized types − seminoma, interstitial cell tumour and Sertoli cell tumour; more than one histological type may be present in a single testis. It is now well documented that the incidence of tumours is significantly higher in retained testes than in normally descended gonads, for which reason removal of the undescended testis is advisable before neoplastic change is likely to occur. In any unilateral cryptorchid in which the testis is abdominally retained neoplasia should be considered in the differential diagnosis of several clinical syndromes. Tumours have also been reported in the testes of pseudohermaphrodites.

Seminoma

This usually occurs in only one testicle and is quite common in normally descended gonads. It often attains a considerable size, a dimension of up to 10 cm being not uncommon. It is nearly always benign and not endocrinologically active, hence the clinical signs are usually related solely to its size. It is surprising how many dogs are presented with a pendulous lesion of considerable size which must cause some discomfort from sheer weight and which certainly mechanically interferes with gait, and yet which owners claim not to have noticed until very recently. The mass is usually painless on pressure and is of firm, regular consistence; the overlying scrotal skin is often not adherent but in some cases adhesions and even ulceration do arise, probably due to trauma when lying.

   Treatment is surgical and is usually quite straightforward. There is usually a greatly increased blood supply via much enlarged spermatic vessels and care is needed in haemostasis; the use of double ligatures or a figure-of-eight pattern in a single ligature is to be recommended for both artery and vein. The testicle can usually be shelled out of the scrotal skin with ease but if adhesions exist there is ample skin available to permit amputation of part of the scrotum; it is often wise to trim away excess skin even in non-adherent cases. The usual care should be paid to ligation of the vessels accompanying the cremaster muscle in the tunica vaginalis as these can be a source of undesirable haemorrhage.

Some clinicians recommend removal of the contralateral testicle whenever a neoplastic testis is removed. If the second gonad seems normal on careful palpation, however, it would seem preferable to leave it in situ rather than render the patient a neuter; this point is arguable. Metastasis is very rare and for all practical purposes seminomas can be regarded as benign.

Interstitial cell tumours

These are probably the least clinically significant. They seldom attain much size although they may be palpable as a nodule of alien consistence (usually firmer) in the testicle tissue and are often unsuspected until a testicle is removed for some reason or at postmortem examination. Endocrinological activity and metastasis are rare. Interstitial cell tumours frequently coexist with other lesions. Diagnosis of the tumour type will only be made histologically and it is rarely that surgery will be directed to the removal of an interstitial cell tumour as such.

Sertoli cell tumour

This is by far the most clinically significant of the canine testicular tumours as it is frequently endocrinologically active and can produce a wide range of sex hormones from androgen to oestrogen. It seldom attains much size in descended testes and is often only diagnosed by deduction from the clinical signs shown; it can, however, become a very large mass in an abdominally retained gonad. It occasionally metastasizes.

Clinical syndromes associated with Sertoli cell tumours

Evidence of sex inversion

The dog shows penile atrophy, a flabby pendulous prepuce and enlargement of the nipples; there may be frank gynaecomastia with development of palpable mammary tissue and even mastitis. Often the owner seeks advice because the dog has become sexually attractive to other males which is a source of nuisance and embarrassment as the patient may become as attractive as a bitch in oestrus.

Skin changes

The dog may show hair loss which can be regarded as hormonal alopecia; this may be bilaterally symmetrical or may mainly affect the posterior dorsum. Secondary bacterial infection is common.

Prostatic changes

Due to tumour secretion of 'female' hormones there may be symptoms of urethral haemorrhage or of urinary problems like dysuria, probably associated with squamous metaplasia of prostatic epithelium. Focal squamous metaplasia of renal tubular epithelium may also be observed at postmortem examination (Lindberg et al., 1970).

Signs suggestive of an intra-abdominal mass

Neoplasia of an abdominally retained testicle should be considered as a differential diagnosis in any patient which is cryptorchid, in which the gonad(s) are not palpable in the inguinal region and in which the presenting signs such as discomfort when lying, or even mildly obstructive signs such as inappetance and vomiting cannot easily be diagnosed as referable to an obvious cause. Laparotomy is to be recommended in such circumstances even if an abdominal mass is not palpable.

Treatment of Sertoli cell tumours is by removal of the effected testis whether it is scrotal, inguinal or abdominal. Results are usually most gratifying with normal male status being restored and resolution of skin changes as a rule within 6-12 weeks of surgery.

Tissue elements found in large abdominal masses are many and varied in addition to the neoplastic testicle; cyst cavities and even bony metaplasia have been recognized.

Orchitis

Inflammation of the testis or testes may occur acutely with obvious symptoms of clinical illness, or insidiously and asymptomatically but with loss of function. Because of their intimate attachment inflammation usually involves the testis and epididymis simultaneously, producing orchi-epididymitis and may extend to the serosal cavity as peri-orchitis. Inflammation of the spermatic cord may also be concurrent with particularly damaging effects upon the testis likely in the event of vascular disturbance.

Orchitis is therefore seldom a clearly demarcated condition, and the consequence of inflammation may relate to damage in any or all structures. Functional obstruction of the epididymis and adhesion to the scrotal wall are, for example, relatively common. Although more commonly unilateral than bilateral, the continuing function of the contralateral organ may be impaired due to the secondary effects of transient local or systemic hyperthermia and possibly auto-immune reaction to exposure of the immune system of the dog to foreign spermatozoal antigens in the inflamed testis. These effects are sometimes initially difficult to assess because of the time lag in maturation of spermatozoa during passage through the epididymis, but in man their viability is known to be adversely affected even by the relative hyperthermia associated with inguinal herniation of abdominal viscera.

In the acute case symptoms are of swelling, heat and progressive discomfort, sometimes with systemic illness. The subject may seek the comfort of cool surfaces and may aggravate the situation by excessive licking of the swollen scrotum with resultant oedema and ulceration and a worsening prognosis. The testis is usually swollen and of firm texture with the epididymis also enlarged, especially caudally. The serosal cavity may also be tensely distended with accumulated fluid.

Examination is naturally resented and it is usually impossible to collect semen samples however useful their examination may be deemed to be.

In the chronic case the organ is atrophied and fibrotic, often irregularly contracted and of firm texture and adherent to the scrotum. A variety of pathological changes including abscesses, spermatoceles and granulomas may be present and result in acute flare-ups with episodes of pain and pyrexia. Aetiology of orchitis is often obscure. It may, of course, follow obvious trauma, but less obviously it may follow general body trauma when abdominal pressure changes may have caused retrograde flushing of urine or prostatic fluid into the vas deferens. Acute prostatic inflammation may also cause orchiepididymitis by the same route, but occasionally infection is of apparently septicaemic origin.

Peri-orchitis may also occur as a sequel to generalized intraperitoneal inflammation, although this appears to be of relatively rare occurrence.

In the United Kingdom there are no canine diseases of which orchitis is an especially notable feature, but where *Br. canis* is endemic, and venereally transmitted, both acute orchi-epididymitis with peri-orchitis and chronic orchi-epididymitis are associated with the infection in the male. Insidious chronic orchi-epididymitis may also be associated with canine distemper infection in the adult dog.

Various bacterial infections including staphylococci, streptococci, *E. coli* and *Proteus vulgaris* are routinely encountered. Management of these cases presents problems. The untreated acute case may abscessate and drain through the scrotum, and in order to preserve the contralateral testis from irreversible thermal damage it is preferable that the affected testis be removed surgically in order to minimize local tissue reaction. Such cases are, in fact, generally unresponsive to routine medical therapy.

Treatment of the acute case presents problems in all circumstances, but especially when retention of fertility is considered to be of paramount importance. In particular it has to be borne in mind that drug therapy which is successful in the control of the acute episode may permanently impair spermatogenesis. High-dose corticosteroid therapy must therefore be avoided. Selection of an antibiotic must, where possible, be on the basis of sensitivity swabbing, or a broad-spectrum agent must be used. In cases of peri-orchitis accumulated fluid may be drawn off hypodermically from the scrotal cavity and it may also be logical to attempt to ensure scrotal cooling in order to protect against the effects of local hyperthermia. In cases of lack of response, surgical removal of the affected testis may be considered preferable to the hazard of total loss of function bilaterally.

A preventative approach to the treatment of the adult human male at high risk from orchitis associated with mumps virus is to induce a state of suppression of spermatogenesis by the administration of oestrogens. Although apparently ineffective when symptoms have commenced, this treatment administered in anticipation of infection has proved valuably protective with a high rate of return to normal testicular function. It would be difficult to assess the potential of such treatment in the dog, except possibly in cases of endemic *Br. canis* infection. However, under such circumstances an eradication policy should logically be practised.

In cases of chronic orchi-epididymitis symptoms of subfertility or infertility may be the initial presenting signs and treatment will be limited to the removal of the damaged testes should they be considered a continuing source of infection. It is likely that many cases of chronic testicular damage will remain unnoticed in non-breeding animals.

EPIDIDYMIS

Anatomy of epididymis

Comparatively large in the dog, the epididymis comprises a much folded tubular structure supported by connective tissue. This provides storage for spermatozoa while adding elements of seminal fluid by secretion of its lining epithelium, as the fluid moves slowly through towards the vas deferens.

Pathology of epididymis

Inflammation

The involvement of the epididymis in orchi-epididymitis and peri-orchiepididymitis has already been considered (p. 129). Specific lesions of the epididymis are rarely reported in the dog, but in man and bull sperm granulomas and spermatoceles are relatively common.

Congenital lesions

Aplasia of the epididymis and associated vas deferens has been occasionally described in various breeds of dog (Copland and Maclachlan, 1976), and in some cases the deficiency has been palpable during routine examination of subjects presenting azoospermia. There is no information available on the heritability of this condition and it is, of course, likely that many cases pass undiagnosed in non-breeding animals. Also, except by direct examination of affected parts, the diagnosis cannot be confirmed, and in some cases may, in fact, relate to deficiency only of the internal tubular structure which is not readily discernible to naked-eye examination.

SPERMATIC CORD

Anatomy of spermatic cord

The contents of the cord, invested by a serosal sheath evaginated from the serosal lining of the scrotal cavity, are the cremaster muscle, the ductus (vas) deferens, the arterial and autonomic nervous supply to scrotal contents and the venous and lymphatic drainage from them.

Arteries are the cremasteric branch of the deep femoral artery, the ductus deferens branch of the urogenital division of the internal iliac, supplying the ductus and epididymis, and the internal spermatic supplying the testis and to some extent the scrotum.

Lymphatic drainage is slightly variable, but unremarkable, and venous drainage complements arterial supply except for the presence of an extensive pampiniform plexus around all other cord vessels at the level of the lower end of the ductus. Nerves are autonomic arising from the pelvic plexus to supply smooth musculature of the scrotum, testis and ductus deferens. The testicular supply, via the external spermatic nerve, comprises sympathetic nerves to blood vessels and smooth muscle tissues. Parasympathetic fibres probably innervate only the musculature of the epididymis and ductus deferens.

The ductus (vas) deferens is functionally a continuation of the duct of epididymis running from the caudal epididymal attachment to the penile urethra. Its relatively simple mucosal lining has no apparent secretory function and its smooth muscular wall is arranged in three layers. There is no ampulla of the duct at its urethral point of attachment, as seen in some species, and both left and right ducts are seen to come into close apposition before penetrating the prostate gland, which masks their dual slit openings into the urethra.

Pathology of spermatic cord

Torsion of spermatic cord

Torsion, with consequent vascular engorgement and infarction of the related testis, is occasionally reported. The majority of cases have involved abdominally retained testes of cryptorchids in which there has been evidence of testicular neoplastic change (Pearson and Kelly, 1975). In the few cases reported in normally descended testes (Young, 1979) dramatic diagnostic changes have not been immediately apparent in the scrotum, most subjects initially exhibiting symptoms of malaise including anorexia, emesis, reduced exercise tolerance and mild pyrexia, but with eventual development of scrotal oedema and palpable testicular swelling. In descended testes, neoplasia has not been a recorded feature of the syndrome, but there has been some recorded evidence of rupture of the scrotal ligament. Presenting signs associated with rotation of an inguinal or intra-abdominal testis are various, some relating more directly to the effects of hormonal changes evoked by neoplastic developments within the testis prior to torsion of its spermatic cord. Thus, in the series reported by Pearson and Kelly (1975), symptoms of dysuria, haematuria and in a few cases flow of fresh blood from the urethra were considered to relate to prostatic disease resulting from the presence of Sertoli cell tumours. Detailed histopathological examination of tissues in that series also gave rise to the suggestion that in some cases torsion might occur gradually over a period of days or weeks, rather than abruptly. The extent of torsion as measured by the number of rotations was also seen to vary.

The most obvious presenting symptoms relating to torsion were posterior stiffness and pain, with reluctance to stand or exercise and an associated anorexia and general malaise. In some cases abdominal palpation confirmed the presence of a painful mass.

In all cases involving abdominally retained testicles there remains an element of doubt in diagnosis because of the confusing similarity of signs presented by uncomplicated neoplasia. Thus laparotomy and direct examination of the spermatic cord is necessary for confirmation.

The aetiology of the condition, especially when affecting normal, descended testicles, is unclear. Trauma and overvigorous exercise have been hypothesized although many recorded subjects have been of mature years. Occurrence in retained testes is relatively easier to understand, in particular as a sequel to the development of uneven and unbalancing neoplastic enlargement. Treatment in all cases is orchidectomy.

The likelihood of occurrence of this potentially fatal condition in the cryptorchid is a clear indication for advocacy of the early surgical removal of retained testes.

The place of castration in veterinary practice

Neither author favours the routine castration of male dogs as a means of controlling numbers. The majority of male dogs, if properly managed, are not unduly highly sexed and adapt to a celibate existence without overt evidence of frustration. The majority of cases of benign hypertrophy of the prostate occur in dogs which have had no sexual experience, but it is probable that the presumed prophylactic effects of mating would only prevail in dogs in regular use, i.e. stud dogs.

Puppies castrated before puberty are subject to similar undesirable changes as are bitches spayed too early, but these effects appear to be more marked in the male. Gross overweight is common and the lack of personality and normal canine social behaviour is even more noticeable in the male, mainly because the male dog is so active in social and territory marking activities. Furthermore, cases are known of castrated males which have been or have become extremely vicious; a somewhat surprising observation. Another surprising side-effect is the development of signs of sex inversion, i.e. attractiveness to other males, which are severe enough to warrant consideration of euthanasia. Whilst these effects are admittedly uncommon it is prudent to mention the possibility to owners considering castration of their dogs. On the other hand it must in fairness be stated that dogs castrated after puberty are less affected by such changes and that people using dogs for work of certain types, e.g. filming, strongly advocate the procedure. It is possible that dogs which work regularly, physically and/or mentally are less affected by a neuter state than the average household pet.

Castration is a very rewarding technique when used as a therapeutic measure. Indications include:

1. Benign hypertrophy of the prostate. Castration results in rapid and permanent regression in the majority of cases.

2. Testicular tumours. Whether only the affected testis or both testes should be removed is debatable.

3. Removal of ectopic testes at an age when neoplastic change is unlikely to have arisen, i.e. before 6 years in breeds of average longevity.

4. As part of the technique to correct scrotal hernias.

5. May be necessary in some cases of severe scrotal neoplasia.

6. Acute conditions such as torsion of the spermatic cord.

7. It has been suggested as a method of treating the androgen-dependent tumour, circumanal adenoma. However, in a limited clinical trial the effect was found to be transient and thus in no way superior to other methods. Regression of the tumour mass was very rapid after castration but regrowth was evident within 3-6 months.

8. As a means of treating hypersexuality. In such cases very careful enquiry is required to establish that the behavioural and/or physical changes are due to this cause. Dogs which are constantly seeking out oestrous bitches and are away from home often for days at a time are sometimes noted to have an anxious, almost hunted expression, to be in poor bodily condition and to some extent hyperaesthetic; such dogs usually respond extremely well in all respects to castration.

When the behaviour problem complained of is constant roaming or aggression, shown either to people or other dogs, every attempt must be made to establish that there is a sexual aetiology. Both traits may be shown by dogs in which there is no sexual basis and owners are very disappointed when castration fails. When the basis is sexual, results of castration are usually very gratifying.

Under no circumstances should a request to castrate adolescent dogs showing undesirable sexual behaviour be acceded to lightly. Adolescence in the dog is not easily defined either in terms of age or duration. Puberty can occur as early as 5 months (notably in Chows) or as late as 15-18 months (e.g. some hounds), but it is difficult to define the duration of adolescent change, possibly 3-6 months on average. Owners can be advised that when the hitherto very obedient and dependent puppy begins to lose this dependence and even show signs of teenage awkwardness and reaction against training routine, it is probably adolescent and evidence of hypersexuality may be shown. In the majority of cases this subsides within weeks or at most a few months and undesirable habits should be dealt with by appropriate discipline and not too rapid recourse to therapy, either medical or surgical; in some cases therapy is required for a short time.

Technique of castration

The technique of castration is so routine in the veterinary field that only brief mention is warranted here. Clinicians sometimes find that seepage of blood into the scrotum persists, resulting in swelling which is exceedingly slow to resolve, i.e. 6 weeks plus. Many surgeons combat this by repelling the testes into an inguinal site just cranial to the scrotum; however, a scrotal approach, taking very great care over haemostasis, is found to be entirely satisfactory. Haemostasis is achieved by the use of cat-gut (or other absorbable) ligatures applied separately to the spermatic artery and vein, often using a figure-of-eight pattern to preclude slipping. Careful observation has shown that persisting seepage occurs from the vessels accompanying the cremaster muscle and this is controlled separately by appropriate ligation; the cremaster and its vessels can be made easily recognizable by inserting a finger into the incised tunic which makes the structures clearly visible. The technique is much quicker to perform than to describe.

PROSTATE GLAND

Anatomy of prostate

This musculoglandular structure encompasses the neck of the bladder, the terminal ductus deferens and the proximal penile urethra. It has a tough fibrous capsule from which trabeculae penetrate and divide into lobules the compound, tubular glandular tissue and smooth muscle cells which comprise its substance. These glandular structures open, via numerous orifices, into the urethra.

Blood supply is from the urogenital artery and innervation is autonomic although the precise nature of nervous control is enigmatic. Stimulation of the sympathetic (hypogastric) nerve supply is reported to provoke secretion which may also be augmented by the administration of para-asympathomimetic drugs. Equally enigmatic is the function of the prostatic secretion. Its alkaline nature suggests that it may usefully neutralize acidic urinary remnants within the urethra, or it may simply function as a flushing agent to assist urethral emptying after ejaculation.

Prostatic pathology

The prostate of the dog is normally sited at the level of the cranial pubic brim, partially encircling the urethra caudal to the bladder and is thus regarded, when normal, as a pelvic organ. Enlargement from any cause may result in either cranial or caudal displacement, in the former case becoming an abdominal viscus often recognizable on palpation. The normal prostate cannot be so palpated, with one qualification, i.e. in some short-legged breeds, particularly Scottish terriers and Welsh corgis, the prostate is recognizable in the posterior abdomen even though no symptoms referable to that organ exist; at the same time it has to be admitted that the gland in such cases is usually larger than average.

In contrast to entire males in most species a high proportion of male dogs remain without sexual experience throughout life, which may be a factor in the development of prostatic disease. Clinical experience suggests that older dogs which have had an active stud life are very seldom presented for problems related to the prostate, but equally so many stud dogs kept by breeders do not reach an old age equivalent to that of many household pets. Most clinical syndromes are related to prostatic enlargement but on rare occasions, to atrophy.

Causes of enlargement include benign hypertrophy, cystic hyperplasia, prostatitis and neoplasia. Occasionally these cannot be differentiated clinically and biopsy is required either by laparotomy or the use of a biopsy needle. Weaver (1977) has reviewed the relatively infrequent use of transperineal needle biopsy techniques in the dog.

Benign hypertrophy

This is an androgen-dependent hypertrophy. It is common in older dogs and may exist asymptomatically. When clinical signs arise they are referable either to defaecation or urinary function. There is a difference of opinion as to which syndrome is commoner, some workers claiming that dysuria is the main presenting sign but experience in general practice suggests that bowel problems predominate.

When the enlarged prostate remains pelvic in position it tends to be displaced more caudally, ventral to the rectum during normal straining efforts at defaecation. As enlargement progresses the prostate exerts pressure on the large bowel acting almost as a valve, and interferes with the progress of faeces through the distal colon and rectum; the result is an increase in straining efforts and eventual tenesmus. The calibre of the faeces often becomes smaller due to pressure obstruction and may reach the stage when they are described as 'pencil stools'. Slowness and incompleteness of bowel emptying may lead to unusually frequent attempts to defaecate. There is little effect on general health in the earlier stages. The role of prostatic hypertrophy in the aetiology of perineal hernia is controversial but the author favours the view that it can be a causal factor.

Urinary signs arise when the prostate becomes more abdominal in position, thus exerting pressure on the urethra as it falls forwards over the pelvic brim. Very occasionally sudden complete urethral obstruction can arise with all the characteristic signs, but more commonly there is a degree of dysuria resulting in increased frequency and straining. If these signs are not detected by the owner a chronic failure of complete emptying of the bladder results with the likelihood of cystitis developing via the residual stale urine.

Diagnosis is made by rectal examination when the bilaterally symmetrical enlargement can easily be recognized. In early cases the gland may be in the normal position when examined, only being displaced caudally during straining; in advanced cases the prostate has often attained a permanently pelvic position and may be felt within 1–1½ in. of the anus.

The enlargement of benign hypertrophy is characteristically bilaterally symmetrical, firm and smooth, not painful on digital pressure and contains no fluid-filled areas, whereas these are present in the rarer condition of cystic hyperplasia.

Wheaton et al. (1979) report sperm viability to be unimpaired in both conditions whereas seminal volume is increased only in the non-cystic subject.

Both surgical and medical treatments are effective although the latter has only a relatively temporary effect and thus needs to be continuous and/or repeated. Castration is usually extremely effective in uncomplicated cases and has the virtue of being permanent and unlikely to be contra-indicated in the age groups concerned. Reduction in the size of the gland occurs remarkably quickly; there is often noticeable diminution at 7 days post-operation and 4 weeks after surgery the prostate has usually returned to a size that is regarded as normal. Prostatectomy is a difficult operation in the dog and is seldom to be recommended.

Medical therapy is by the use of the anti-androgenic effects of the female sex hormones, oestradiol and stilboestrol, or by the use of a specific anti-androgen, in particular delmadinone. Dosage recommendations for the synthetic stilboestrol diproprionate are 3–5 mg daily by mouth or 15 mg by implantation. Oestradiol 10 or 20 mg implants can be used similarly and treatment repeated as required. Delmadinone acetate by intramuscular or subcutaneous routes is used on a sliding scale at 1·5–2·0 mg/kg up to 10 kg body weight, 1·0–1·5 mg/kg between 10 and 20 kg body weight, and thereafter at 1·0 mg/kg. Repeat treatment is at 3-weekly intervals unless relative non-response indicates the need for more frequent dosage.

Prostatitis

This is less common than benign hypertrophy but does occur regularly. Although it is seldom seen in young dogs it does arise in a somewhat lower age group and is associated with systemic signs.

Clinical signs are not always easy to recognize nor are they easily described by the owner, so great care in history taking is required. There is usually some evidence of general malaise such as raised temperature, decreased appetite and lessened activity. More characteristic signs are referable to the existence of an inflamed and probably painful viscus, and include unusual posture when sitting down or lying and a changed gait which may be due to straddling of the hindlegs or a somewhat arched back and very cautious movement.

On rectal examination the prostate is usually decidedly enlarged, is painful on digital pressure and the tissue is less smooth than in hypertrophy. The enlargement may or may not be symmetrical. When local abscess formation has occurred it is often possible to recognize the fluctuating or even frankly fluid-filled focus. In such cases fever is usually a prominent feature.

Microscopic examination of urine in cases of prostatitis will usually demonstrate leucocytes, pus cells and bacteria, but as similar findings will be present in some cases of cystitis differentiation will have to be based largely on recognition of changes in the organ involved, i.e. either painful enlargement (prostate) or a thickened, probably contracted, bladder. It is difficult to obtain a specimen of urine which can be relied upon accurately to reflect the level of infection in the urinary tract.

Bacteriological examination is desirable. However, therapy should not be delayed as early treatment may prevent localization with pus development. A broad-spectrum antibacterial agent should be utilized at once and change can be made to the indicated drug following sensitivity tests.

Although there may be symptomatic improvement fairly quickly, the changes in the prostate follow much more slowly and progress must be monitored by rectal examination repeated at suitable intervals as dictated by the general condition of the patient.

The cautious use of small doses of oestrogens and corticosteroids has, in some cases, appeared to be effective in reducing the size of the gland but these must only be introduced following and combined with effective antibacterial treatment. In some patients considerable prostate enlargement persists even after objective signs have disappeared. Prognosis in prostatitis cases is always guarded.

Abscess formation is always a serious development as localized accumulations of pus do not usually respond adequately to antibacterial therapy unless drainage can be provided. Various techniques designed to provide such drainage have been attempted but none has been consistent enough in results to warrant its inclusion in routine practice regimes.

Neoplasia

Carcinoma is the commonest type of prostate tumour and although it occurs regularly but infrequently it is far less common than in man. The signs are in no way pathognomonic; it is not unusual for the condition to be unsuspected until metastatic tumours are detected, often in the sublumbar lymph nodes.

Clinical signs are seldom particularly helpful but may include some evidence suggestive of prostatic enlargement or there may be discomfort related to the posterior dorsal region; weight loss occurs as the disease progresses and in this respect differs from other causes of enlarged prostate in which this sign is uncommon. During routine clinical examination enlargement of the more caudal sublumbar lymph nodes is detectable on abdominal palpation and confirmed by rectal examination. Unless there is evidence of generalized enlargement of lymph nodes, e.g. lymphosarcoma, attention should be directed to the prostate. The gland will be found to show enlargement, often asymmetrical, possibly involving only one lobe and the new tissue is usually somewhat nodular or irregular in consistence.

Medical treatment is unlikely to be effective as the tumour is not usually regarded as being hormone-dependent. Once metastasis has occurred a surgical approach is futile and even when it is believed that only the primary tumour exists, operation is not easy and cannot be routinely recommended. As indicated earlier prostatectomy in the dog is not an easy operation due to anatomical factors and prognosis is thus poor. If prostatectomy is to be attempted, the best method is by resection of the prostatic urethra followed by anastamosis of the neck of the bladder to the pelvic urethra caudal to the point of section.

Cysts

These may occur as a cystic hyperplasia apparently unrelated to any other pathological condition of the prostate or may be a complication of prostatitis or neoplasia. The lesion is usually detected during examination when absence of pain on pressure and likewise absence of systemic signs suggest that the fluid-filled area is more likely to be cystic than suppurative. Treatment is seldom undertaken.

Other types of tissue change, usually detected only at postmortem examination, include bony metaplasia; sometimes well-developed plates of bone are found, which it would often seem have caused no clinical signs.

Atrophy

Atrophic changes with fibrosis are very occasionally recognized, often during rectal examination for some other reason. Often the only clinical sign seen is stricture of the urethra with a progressive dysuria. Passage of a catheter becomes difficult at the level of the neck of the bladder and it may not be possible to make a definitive diagnosis without laparotomy. Resection of the affected area of urethra is rarely successful. If fibrosis is suspected the use of corticosteroids at an earlier stage is justified in an attempt to delay the development of urinary obstruction.

Hormone-dependent disease

It has been reported (Reif and Brodey, 1969) that among the 39% of dogs showing Sertoli cell tumour-related feminization, there are some in which secondary prostatic changes may result in symptoms of urinary obstruction and others in which symptoms of persistent flow of urethral blood may occur. In the latter the source of blood is assumed to be prostatic since no urethral lesions have been apparent. Lesions of squamous metaplasia of prostatic epithelium have been described (Lindberg et al., 1976).

URETHRA

Anatomy and physiology

This tubular structure has a dual function, carrying urine and seminal secretion to the penile orifice. Within its prostatic section, extending from the neck of the bladder to the caudal end of the prostate, the longitudinally folded membranous lining of transitional eipthelium is perforated by the twin openings of the vas deferens and the numerous openings of the prostatic ductus. Passing over the caudal pelvic brim and into the spongy, erectile corpus cavernosum urethra, the tubular structure remains similar until, near the orifice, epithelium becomes stratified squamous, continuous with the surface of the glans penis.

Between the prostatic portion and the pelvic brim is a portion of urethra surrounded by a ring of vascularity continuous with the corpus cavernosum urethra, outside which is a layer of glandular tissue overlain by urethral muscle. These, the urethral glands, are the source of the first fraction of the ejaculate.

Urethral musculature, a mixture of smooth longitudinal and striated transverse fibres, is autonomically innervated by the pelvic plexus.

The urethral lumen is considerably distensible by the flattening out of its mucosal folds, except where the corpus cavernosum penis runs within the ventral groove of the penile bone.

Urethral pathology

Congenital abnormalities

These are occasionally encountered, the most frequent being hypospadia, a failure of ventral fusion of the urethra and prepuce along part of its length. This may be encountered in both genetic males and intersexes and is treated by amputation of the distal penile structures. More unusually a dorsal opening may occur. This, epispadia, is attributed to embryonic displacement of cells forming the cloacal membrane and should also be treated surgically. Rarely, conditions of imperforate urethra, urethral agenesis and urethrorectal fistula have been reported.

Urethritis

This may occur as a result of wounds, self-trauma, faulty catheterization, passage of cystic calculi and as a sequel to cystitis. Symptoms will vary according to the severity of inflammation and may be as minor as increased frequency of urination with evidence of stinging discomfort. In some cases haematuria may be noted, particularly at commencement of urination, while in severe cases a haemorrhagic preputial drip may be observed. Extreme urethral discomfort with evidence of obstruction is usually indicative of the lodgement of cystic urinary calculi and rarely occurs due to primary urethritis.

Treatment of urethritis should include routine antibiotic therapy and the oral administration of urinary antiseptics. In recalcitrant cases antibiotic sensitivity swabbing should be performed. In some cases it may be beneficial to increase urine flow by salting the diet or by the administration of diuretics. Aetiological factors, where apparent, should be dealt with routinely. In the case of traumatic wounding of the urethra it is advisable to allow healing by granulation in order to avoid the risk of stricture following unnecessary surgical intervention. In cases of trauma by excessive grooming or self-stimulation appropriate systems of restraint should be instituted.

Urethral obstruction

This is usually associated with urolithiasis in the first instance although it may subsequently be due to fibrous scarring and stricture following urethral surgery or traumatic damage. In cases of stricture formation the onset of obstruction is gradual and treatment can be instituted in anticipation of total obstruction. In cases of urolithiasis, obstruction may be sudden in onset and complete, accompanied by evidence of discomfort and distress and, in the untreated case, the development of uraemia or urethral rupture. Lodgement of calculi may be at any site, but the commonest is the caudal end of the os penis at which point distensibility of the urethra is limited. Confirmation may be obtained by catheterization and it is sometimes possible thus to obtain temporary relief of symptoms by bypassing or gentle repulsion of the calculus. It is, however, not unusual for the urethra to contain several calculi and it is therefore wise to check this situation radiographically before embarking upon corrective surgery.

A technique for the non-surgical removal of calculi from the urethra has been described by Piermattei and Osborne (1971). Using a mixture of sterilized aqueous lubricant (K-Y Jelly — Johnson & Johnson) and sterile water they have evolved techniques of retrograde and antegrade flushing. In both the fluid is initially applied under pressure through the external urethral orifice while digital compression of the pelvic urethra is maintained per rectum. The pressure so created in the closed system effects such distension of the urethral lumen that slight repulsion of the calculus can be achieved. In the case of a calculus which is clearly too large to pass the penile bone, a complete retrograde flush may then be achieved by sudden removal of the pelvic compression. In the case of smaller calculi, antegrade flushing might be achieved by the sudden withdrawal of the catheter from the orifice while maintaining pelvic urethral pressure.

Assuming the success of such manoeuvres, cystotomy for the removal of calculi at source is then performed obviating the necessity for urethral incision, and medical treatments can be instituted to minimize the subsequent formation of calculi.

In the event of failure of these procedures urethrostomy is inevitably necessary though undertaken with reluctance in a stud dog. Often, in cases of firm lodgement of calculi, the selection of surgical site is predetermined, but in some cases it is possible to select a site of incision through which calculi can be removed by retrograde flushing.

The entire length of accessible urethra is surrounded by erectile tissue so that haemorrhage is inevitable, but in the majority of cases it is possible to avoid interference with the highly erectile tissue of the glans. Should incision of this tissue be necessary, a prolonged post-surgical period of sexual abstinence is recommended in order to minimize the risks of severe haemorrhage.

In the selection of the site for incision it is advisable to consider the requirement in a stud dog for flexibility of tissues in the region of the head of the penis so that full penile erection and extrusion can take place without the discomfort that would ensue from adhesions of penile or preputial tissues. A midperineal site might be considered ideal, or else a point midway between the caudal penile bone and the scrotum, care being taken at either location to avoid scrotal involvement.

Since the urethra has a good regenerative capacity it is unnecessary to carry out any wound repair and the placement of sutures is, in fact, contra-indicated on several counts. Effective suturing of the urethral tissue is likely to result in subsequent fibrosis and stenosis, while ineffective suturing will result in the seepage of urine. In the case of an open granulating wound such leakage is of no consequence, but in the case of neat sutures in several layers, leakage may result in urine tracking through the tissues, especially if there is a good degree of adherence of the sutured skin wound. Cases have been seen in which this has resulted in gravitational pooling of urine in pendulous scrotal tissue, with eventual sloughing necessitating surgical resection and castration. It is clearly preferable to tolerate urine dribbling and minor haemorrhage of relatively short duration while allowing natural healing, rather than to risk such postsurgical complications as loss of sexual function. It is difficult to imagine that the degree of fibrosis and stricture which may occur as a result of natural healing is likely to adversely affect the transmission of seminal fluid. In the event of extreme stricture a degree of widening may be achieved by repeated, minor, forced dilatation.

Urethral rupture

This may occur as a result of traumatic incidents, careless catheterization or as a result of obstruction as described. Presenting signs and approaches to treatment will vary according to the site of damage. Because of their inaccessibility, some sites, such as the intrapelvic urethra damaged by pelvic fracture, may best be left to heal naturally, with permanent catheterization ensured to prevent urinary contamination of tissues. At other sites surgical drainage of water-logged tissues might be provided and the urethral wound either sutured or permitted to heal naturally, according to circumstances.

Urethral prolapse

This is uncommon but well documented. Although it may appear as a sequel to excessive straining, it is most commonly the result of sexual overexcitement and self-stimulation by licking. The prolapsed mucosal tissue may vary in length and colour and its rapid replacement is necessary to avoid the risk of oedema and irreversible damage. Replacement by catheterization is sometimes possible and a purse-string suture can be placed for several days to assist retention. Alternatively, resection may be preferred or be necessary in cases of irreversible damage. The apposition of mucosal edges with fine gut sutures is feasible and often successful, but care must be taken in the postsurgical period to avoid sexual excitement or further self-trauma. A combination of ataractic and anti-androgen medical therapy may achieve this. In cases of recurrence castration may eventually become necessary.

PENIS

Anatomy and physiology

Anatomically, the penis of the dog is distinctively different from that of other domestic species. Even in non-erection it is a relatively rigid organ and is firmly anchored to the ventral abdominal wall by the prepuce which, except at the tip, is attached along its entire dorsal edge. There is variation in this respect so that in some dogs the prepuce is so tightly applied to the central abdomen as to appear almost integral, while in others it is more pendulously attached by a longitudinal pedicle of skin that is sometimes almost translucent.

The rigidity of the non-erect organ is to some extent attributable to the presence of a longitudinal penile bone, but also to the fact that much of the substance of the penile shaft is fibrous and relatively non-erectile being, however, overlain at its distal extremity by an extensively developed and highly erectile glans penis, the tumescence of which seems less related to effecting intromission than to achieving the tie. (Grandage, 1972.)

The main body of the penis which is palpable in non-erection comprises two elongated tubes of spongy tissue, the corpora cavernosa penis, of limited erectile capacity, being bounded by firm fibrous capsules and arising with their associated retractor muscles as twin crura from the tuber ischii of the caudal pelvic brim. Palpable in the perineal midline, although overlain by retractor muscles, the joined tubes accommodate in the groove of their ventral connection the penile urethra which is itself here invested with a separate sheath of spongy erectile tissue, the corpus cavernosum urethra, running from its origin as the urethral bulb within the posterior pelvic brim to almost the tip of the penis. At its distal end, the accommodating groove is within the ventral aspect of the penile bone (os penis) which is the forward prolongation of the corpora cavernosa penis finally confluent at a point of approximately halfway along the ventral abdominal portion of the shaft. The penis distal to this point lies within the preputial sheath.

The penile bone is represented at the tip of the penis by a cartilaginous prolongation into the highly erectile pars longa of the glans penis which overlies and envelopes the urethra and os penis, extending back to partially overlie the bulbus glandis, a separate bilaterally distensible erectile organ surrounding the caudal half of the os penis and arising as distension from the spongy corpus cavernosum urethra. In non-erection the bulbus glandis may be represented by barely perceptible symmetrical swellings. In the excited young dog these swellings may become very noticeably distended, even during periods of non-sexual excitement, without full penile erection occurring. In this situation the distensions may mistakenly be the cause of owner concern and may even be misdiagnosed as testicular tissue in cryptorchid subjects.

Arterial blood supply to the penis is chiefly via the internal pudendal branch of the visceral division of the internal iliac artery, with a lesser supply from anastomosis with the external pudendal. The venous drainage pattern is complex and the control of blood flow in the attainment and maintenance of erection dependent upon it. This process is described in detail by Miller et al. (1964).

Innervation is from the sacral plexus of sympathetic and parasympathetic nerves via paired pudendal and pelvic nerves. The pudendal nerve provides the dorsal penile nerve and sensory innervation of the glans as well as perineal innervation and motor supply to the penile retractor muscles. The pelvic nerves supply sensory and visceral innervation to the intrapelvic portion of the urogenital tract and the hypogastric nerves are responsible for ejaculation and prostatic secretion.

Penile pathology

Congenital abnormalities

Congenital abnormalities of the penis are relatively uncommon. The most obvious have been dealt with in consideration of the urethra and of intersex conditions (p. 189). Less dramatic deformities may pass unnoticed since the majority of dogs are not used for breeding and their genital organs are consequently rarely subjected to close scrutiny. Occasionally slight deformity of the shaft may be encountered which is attributable to malformation of the os penis. This may first be noticed as the cause of clumsy jetting of urine, but is more usually discovered as the cause of persistent misdirection of copulatory effort. Since, except in extreme cases, mating is possible, even unassisted, by dogs with such deformity, it is difficult to assess the frequency of occurrence of this lesion.

Another documented congenital deformity encountered relatively infrequently is persistence of the penile frenulum, a band of fibrous tissue uniting penis and sheath ventrally. The condition has been described in the bull (Ashdown, 1962), in which species rupture normally occurs at puberty, and in the dog (Joshua, 1962), in which the signs noted were similar to those often associated with anal sac conditions, viz. sitting down suddenly and crying out. It is suggested that signs will usually not be noted until puberty, at which stage the intermittent engorgement of the penis described above will cause discomfort. The penis of the younger puppy is seldom examined clinically other than in the diagnosis of dog-pox, so the incidence of persistence is not known. Only the single case recorded was seen in a large number of prepubertal puppies specifically examined for this lesion following Ashdown's (1962) report.

Trauma

Traumatic lesions of the penis are not uncommon as a result of fight wounds, road traffic accidents or sporting activities. These may be relatively trivial or extreme and each case merits individual assessment and treatment. In extreme cases, amputation may be indicated, and when elected is best performed behind the level of the penile bone so that the distensible erectile tissue of the bulbus glandis and glans penis is removed. In case of less radical surgery, the tendency for rapid tumefaction of these tissues during periods of sexual arousal may be an obvious complicating factor, and in order to facilitate wound healing and to reduce the risk of serious haemorrhage, anti-androgen therapy might usefully be considered and a prolonged period of sexual abstinence advised.

The decision of whether or not to suture penetrating wounds will depend in part upon the site and degree of damage. It is probably advisable in order to minimize blood loss to suture wounds in the glans with fine gut while wounds in the spongy shaft should be left to granulate, especially in any case of urethral penetration.

Fracture damage of the os penis

This may present a particular problem especially in small breeds in which logical bone repair procedures such as finger plating or wiring are not feasible. In such cases, insertion of a permanent indwelling urinary catheter might usefully provide support during the healing period during which sexual abstinence should be enforced.

Trauma during copulation

This may also occur and be evident in the immediate post-mating phase as contusions which, however, rapidly disappear. Occasionally slight but insignificant haemorrhage may be noted from the prepuce or the vagina of the bitch.

A persistent contusion of the tip of the penis has been seen in a much used stud dog which broke down and bled copiously at each mating. The lesion was extremely resistant to treatment but eventually responded to local injection of corticosteroid and crystalline penicillin repeated at approximately 10-day intervals. Sexual rest (which had been ineffective per se) for one year was prescribed and the dog returned to service apparently without any recurrence of the lesion.

The significance of such a lesion is related especially to fertility, since blood is considered to be spermicidal and the degree of haemorrhage in such a case into the bitch's vagina might well be inimical to conception.

Infection

Infection might occur due to traumatic damage and should be routinely treated with systemic antibiotic and local wound dressing as indicated.

Dog-pox

This condition has been fully described (Joshua, 1975) and is of very high incidence in the dog population, i.e. over 60%, many cases existing asymptomatically. It is postulated that it may be due to a herpes virus. The penis is the commonest site of lesions, mainly on and caudal to the bulbus glandis. The lesions are papular in type, 1-1·5 mm in diameter, they may occasionally seem to be vesicular (which they are not) and some have a tendency to bleed; histologically they are simply aggregations of lymphocytes.

Clinical signs include irritation and abnormal preputial discharge; surprisingly, haemorrhage is not a common sign. Evidence of irritation is sometimes difficult to interpret and may even suggest anal sac pathology; more usually it is shown by sudden excessive licking or nibbling, often in a somewhat random manner, at the hindquarters, scrotal area and inside thighs.

It is essential to extrude the penis completely and to reflect it posteriorly out of the sheath in order to examine properly the predilection site. Since lesions are also found in the lower bowel and conjunctiva these mucosae should also be examined, especially as bowel lesions are liable to cause the most distressing signs.

The mode of transmission is not known but it is certainly not solely venereal as many dogs with no sexual contact have lesions as do pre-pubertal puppies. Lesions have been detected as early as 4 months of age.

Treatment regrettably is non-specific and seldom results in the total disappearance of lesions although symptoms often decrease considerably. The antiviral agent idoxuridine is not practicable on the grounds of its method of application and response on a mucosal surface. The author has used it in one case, quite ineffectually and with some significant tissue damage which did eventually resolve spontaneously but was unacceptable in degree.

The topical use of antibacterial agents appears to have some palliative effect and reduces preputial discharge. Cauterization of lesions with a solution of silver nitrate not exceeding 5% in strength and rapidly control-led by saline is well tolerated and again appears to be symptomatically effective. Intramammary preparations of antibacterial agents are a very useful method of application; they may be introduced into the preputial orifice and then gently massaged backwards along the sheath.

Symptoms are curiously intermittent in intensity, many infected dogs showing no signs for weeks or months and then having an episode of severe irritation. Prognosis is inevitably guarded as to the complete remission of signs.

Transmissible venereal tumour (TVT)

This has already been discussed as it occurs in the bitch (p. 27). The tumour is probably commoner in the male owing to its more promiscuous behaviour when not properly controlled. Again it is most commonly seen in large seaports and is found in dogs recently released from quarantine.

The site of tumour formation is the mucous membrane of the glans penis; any site from the tip to the bulb can be involved, although it is uncommon behind the bulb.

The clinical sign is almost invariably preputial haemorrhage which is quite unrelated to urination; the general health of the dog is rarely affect-ed. Examination of the penis reveals the lesion which, as in the bitch, is proliferative, has a roughened surface and bleeds easily; it also tends to develop in an annular fashion and may eventually involve the whole circumference of the penis.

Diagnosis is virtually obvious since there are no real differentials; histology is pathognomonic and an impression smear, stained by simple methods, can readily be used in practice as the hepatoid cells are easily recognized.

Treatment is surgical, by resection of the tumour-bearing mucous membrane. Operation is straightforward and surprisingly large areas of mucosa can be removed; provided the section is made in healthy tissue, recurrence at the site should not occur and metastasis is uncommon. The only postoperative complication seen has been paraphimosis due to the constriction produced by the suture line apposing the incised mucosal edges, but even this usually resolves within a reasonable period of time. Results are usually gratifying.

PREPUCE

Anatomy of prepuce

This tubular sheath covers approximately half the length of the non-erect penis, virtually the entire length of bony penis, including the pars longa glandis and anterior portions of bulbus glandis, lying within its cavity. The outer surface is of skin, continuous with that of the ventral abdomen, and the inner of smooth, stratified squamous epithelium continuous at the fornix with the epithelial surface of the bulbus glandis and penis. Strips of preputial muscle extend to the prepuce from the region of the xiphoid cartilage and probably assist retention of the prepuce over the glans. They may also prevent the tip of the non-erect organ from hanging too far from the abdominal wall.

Sensory innervation of the inner surface is pudendal via the dorsal nerve of the penis while parietal surfaces have ilio-inguinal and iliohypogastric innervation.

Preputial pathology

Congenital abnormalities

Various congenital abnormalities of the prepuce occur and are usually recognized during early puppyhood. Possibly the commonest is a too small orifice which may be only large enough to permit the passage of single drops of urine with resulting retention of urine within the sheath, constant dribbling of urine and general soiling. This is usually recognized when puppies are only a few weeks old and remedial surgery is required at an early stage. Less severe cases may not cause any interference with urination but may make complete extrusion and withdrawal of the penis difficult during attempted mating.

Treatment is by plastic surgery, usually comprising incision of the ventral edge of the preputial orifice followed by very careful suturing of the incised edges of skin to mucous membrane on each side; absorbable suture material is usually adequate as healing is rapid. Care must be taken not to enlarge the orifice too much; too long an incision results in the tip of the penis being visible whenever the dog is recumbent and, even though desiccation of the penile tip is not common, many owners find the situation aesthetically unacceptable.

Occasionally the sheath is not fully developed and does not adequately enclose the penis. Although adverse effects are rare the condition is often not acceptable to owners and in severe cases euthanasia may be requested.

Dog-pox

Although the penis is the commoner site of lesions these do occasionally extend onto the mucosa of the prepuce, usually caudal to the bulbus glandis. The only significance of this is that the penis itself may be free of lesions thus leading to a negative diagnosis, whereas if a finger is introduced into the prepuce the lesions can be palpated on the preputial mucosa. Involvement of this site usually causes obvious signs of irritation.

Haemorrhage from the prepuce

This is a fairly common clinical sign which can arise from a variety of causes. Differential diagnosis is essential to determine the source of bleeding hence very careful history taking and clinical examination is required. It is surprising how often cases are referred for investigation when a thorough examination at average GP level would have determined the cause.

The following are some points to be considered: relationship of the bleeding to urination; if related, is it early in urination, distributed throughout urine or passed at the end of micturition? Is there any evidence of systemic signs, with special reference to polydipsia/polyuria? If bleeding is unrelated to urination, is it intermittent and, if so, how frequent; if not, is it continuous and, if so, how copious? Does it appear to be pure blood? Is it related to sexual excitement?

Possible sites of bleeding include the bladder, the prostate, the urethra, the penis and the prepuce.

Bladder

The haemorrhage is usually related to urination and, more commonly, towards later urination (it cannot be described as at the end of urination in the male dog). Differential diagnosis will include cystitis, with or without calculus formation, neoplasms or other bleeding points unrelated to these.

Prostate

This is a site not always considered if there is no obvious sign suggestive of prostatic disease. If there is no obvious alternative source of blood, rectal examination of the prostate should be performed when an enlargement may be recognized. Castration in such cases is usually effective. Bleeding due to squamous metaplasia of prostatic epithelium may occur secondary to Sertoli cell tumour development of the testis.

Urethra

This is not a common site of haemorrhage but occasionally blood is passed in the urine in long-standing cases of partial obstruction by urethral calculi.

Penis

Traumatic lesions sustained in fights or street incidents or during coitus may bleed and are usually obvious. TVT causes preputial haemorrhage. Occasionally ulceration into a surface blood vessel of the glans occurs. Although dog-pox lesions may appear haemorrhagic they seldom cause blood to emerge from the prepuce.

Prepuce

The usual cause will be traumatic lesions. It is sometimes possible to determine at examination whether the blood is actually emerging via the urethra or is external to it, but sometimes this requires prolonged observation in order to differentiate.

REFERENCES

Arthur G. H. (1956) Fellowship thesis. Royal College of Veterinary Surgeons, London.

Ashdown R. R. (1962) Persistence of the penile frenulum in young bulls. *Vet. Rec.* **74**, 1464–1468.

Ashdown R. R. (1963) The diagnosis of cryptorchidism in young dogs: a review of the problem. *J. Small Anim. Pract.* **4**, 261–263.

Copland M. D. and Maclachlan N.L. (1976) Aplasia of epididymis and vas deferens in the dog. *J. Small Anim. Pract.* **17**, 443–449.

Grandage J. (1972) The erect dog penis: A paradox of flexible rigidity. *Vet. Rec.* **91**, 141–147.

Joshua J. O. (1962) Persistence of the penile frenulum in a dog. *Vet. Rec.* **74**, 1550.

Joshua J. O. (1975) 'Dog pox'. *Vet. Rec.* **96**, 300–302.

Lindberg R., Jonsson O.-J. and Kasstrom H. (1976) Sertoli cell tumours associated with feminization, prostatitis and squamous metaplasia of the renal tubular epithelium. *J. Small Anim. Pract.* **17**, 451.

Miller M. E., Christensen G. C. and Evans H. E. (1964) *Anatomy of the Dog.* Philadelphia, Saunders.

Pearson H. and Kelly D. F. (1975) Testicular torsion in the dog: a review of 13 cases. *Vet. Rec.* **97**, 200.

Piermattei D. L. and Osborne C. A. (1971) Nonsurgical removal of calculi from the urethra of male dogs. *J. Am. Vet. Med. Assoc.* **159**, 1755–1757.

Reif J. S. and Brodey R. S. (1969) The relationship between cryptorchidism and canine testicular neoplasia. *J. Am. Vet. Med. Assoc.* **155**, 2005–2010.

Weaver A. D. (1977) Transperineal punch biopsy of the canine prostate gland. *J. Small Anim. Pract.* **18**, 573.

Wheaton L. G., De Klerk D. P., Strandberg J. D. et al. (1979) Relationship of seminal volume to size and disease of the prostate gland in the beagle. *Am. J. Vet. Res.* **40**, 1325–1328.

Young A. C. B. (1979) Two cases of intrascrotal torsion of a normal testicle. *J. Small Anim. Pract.* **20**, 229.

Chapter 12

Infertility

Introduction

Throughout this book reference has been made to factors relevant to the disruption of normal reproductive processes. Such factors are here discussed under the collective title of infertility. Classification of the causes of infertility is arbitrary and they are discussed here as anatomical, physiological, infectious and psychological causes considered separately in the female and the male as appropriate.

Under field conditions such classification may initially be impossible and it may even be equivocal that an infertility problem exists. In the case of certain diseases, for example *Brucella canis* infection on a kennel basis, the situation may actually be of subfertility, or low-level attainment, and it may be that similar patterns exist in relation to other diseases as yet unrecognized. Under some circumstances a low level of kennel attainment is more readily noticeable to an outside observer than to a kennel keeper habituated to low litter numbers, neonatal deaths, repeat breeders, etc.

FEMALE-RELATED INFERTILITY

Anatomical causes

Congenital anomalies

In extreme cases there may be ovarian agenesis with total absence of sexual maturity and oestrous cyclic habit. In the event of absence of pro-oestrus within an age considered reasonable for the breed, investigation may be initiated either medically or surgically. The medical approach is as outlined for the initiation of oestrus (pp. 38, 39) and the response to injection with FSH may also be monitored by measurement of blood levels of oestrogens as an indicator of stimulated ovarian activity. In the event of lack of this measurement facility or the absence of visible response to medical stimulation, laparotomy may be performed for direct examination of the ovaries, or techniques of laparoscopy may be preferred (Doyle, 1951). In either event, the position of the ovarian fat bursa obstructs viewing.

In some such cases of cyclic absence in apparent females, direct investigation may reveal the animal to be pseudo-hermaphrodite. In the rarer true hermaphrodite the presence of male and female gonadal tissue may result in an apparently normal oestrous cyclic habit. Congenital abnormality of the Fallopian tubes, in particular agenesis, is not easily diagnosed other than by detailed postmortem examination, since limitations of direct in vivo examination are as described for ovaries. Chemical methods of determining tubal patency, for example the phenol sulphon-ephthalein test (Kessy and Noakes, 1979), may presumably be adaptable for use in the bitch, but await evaluation. Techniques of combined tubal insufflation and salpingography appear not to have been applied (Sweeney, 1958) and indeed few investigations of individual infertility are taken thus far.

Such congenital anatomical abnormalities of the uterus as unilateral aplasia, though recorded, need not necessarily impair fertility. Congenital anatomical abnormalities of the vagina largely impair fertility by virtue of obstructed intromission, and it is possible that, following their surgical correction or by means of artificial insemination, pregnancy might result. As stated previously, accumulating evidence of a familial incidence of such abnormalities is both disturbing and apparently significant in one breed (the Chow) in which 'non-breeder' bitches are numerous.

The condition of vestibulovaginal stenosis recently reviewed (Holt and Sayle, 1981) in the context of a syndrome of vulval pruritus, urinary frequency and a degree of urinary incontinence, may similarly present a barrier to intromission. It is uncertain to what extent the condition occurs and it is likely that only relatively severe cases present the problem, in which case no treatment should be offered to effect a mating and pregnancy.

In some of these cases well-developed hymenal tissue has been noted at the level of the vestibulovaginal junction and there are occasional reports (Furneaux, 1979) of the presence of imperforate hymen presenting an obstruction of vaginal drainage. It is difficult to assess the frequency of such occurrence since the prevalence of the lay habit of 'breaking the bitch down' digitally relates to the mistaken assumption of direct analogy with human hymenal anatomy.

Tension in the region of the cingulum obstructing intromission or causing bitch resistance is usually rapidly responsive to medical treatment with chlorpromazine. Although some veterinarians do not find it necessary to resort to surgical incision of obstructing tissue, such surgical 'dilatation' is fairly commonplace.

Congenital vulval infantilism, probably more properly considered a physiological defect, is unresponsive to chlorpromazine therapy. In the event of intromission occurring, considerable distress to the male may result from the lack of distensibility of the tissues.

Acquired anomalies

Post-inflammatory adhesion within ovarian bursae and Fallopian tubes might rarely present as the cause of infertility, though not as part of a well-recognized disease syndrome as in some species. In suspected cases, techniques for the establishment of diagnosis are as described for congenitally acquired defects.

Acquired anatomical defects of the uterus are unlikely to present as the cause of infertility, since postsurgical healing of canine uterine wounds is good. Such adhesions with abdominal viscera as may occur rarely present problems, even during parturition.

Acquired cervical scarring and distortion following obstetrical procedures may presumably obstruct sperm transport, but this is difficult to substantiate except by detailed postmortem examination. However, the increasing sophistication of vaginal endoscopic techniques may result in diagnosis by this means.

Fibrous scarring in the region of the cingulum as a result of previous rupture due to intromission or careless digital examination may present a barrier to intromission and cause bitch discomfort. Simple surgical correction may be performed. Postsurgical scarring following episiotomy for the removal of polypi or resection of hypertrophied vestibulovaginal tissues rarely results in difficulties, though a surgical reduction in the vulval aperture may do so.

Vaginal polypi and neoplasia need not necessarily present barriers to intromission, fertilization and pregnancy, but may impede parturition.

Physiological causes

The complexity of hormonal events governing sexual function is such that the wonder is that so few malfunctions occur. Certainly, hormonal treatments favoured for their medical control are relatively gross and imprecise.

Abnormality of oestrous cycle

1. *Absence of oestrous cyclic activity or delayed puberty*

In clinically healthy animals exhibiting no other endocrinological malfunction, the cause of this condition is enigmatic. Techniques for the induction of oestrus and ovulation have been described (p. 38), but it is arguable that they should be routinely employed in such circumstances.

Because of the uncertainty of the effect of vitamin and mineral imbalances it is worthwhile in such cases paying attention to dietary intake. Bitches fed exclusively on compound maintenance rations may benefit from the substitution of a more mixed dietary intake of good quality. A clinical observation in support of this suggestion is the resumption of cyclic activity by bitches exhibiting prolonged anoestrus some weeks after the commencement of supplementation of their compound maintenance rations by the addition of raw meat.

It is very difficult to decide what should properly be called abnormality in view of the wide limits of assumed normality. There is considerable breed and individual variation in the age at which a first cycle occurs. The majority of bitches have been on heat before one year of age but in some breeds, especially hounds, it is common for the first cycle to occur between 15 and 18 months of age. It is probably justifiable to consider any bitch which has not been on heat by 18–24 months as abnormal, although hormonal therapy to induce a cycle is almost certainly better delayed for a further 6–12 months. There is no useful purpose in attempting induction in bitches not intended for breeding as there is no evidence that the very delayed onset of cycling is detrimental to health. In the event of failure of medical therapy, the possibility of ovarian agenesis should be investigated.

2. Prolonged anoestrus between cycles

Whilst the average periodicity is 6-monthly, quite a degree of variation between breeds, individuals and even in a given individual should not necessarily be regarded as an abnormality requiring treatment. Nine- to twelve-month intervals are quite common. It is also well recognized that following breeding the next heat may be delayed some 4–8 weeks beyond the 6-month date. Intervals of 12 months or more occurring in a bitch which has hitherto had relatively regular heats of normal intensity are probably evidence of deficiency of ovarian function, whether at ovarian or pituitary level. On the other hand, some bitches which have hitherto been regular seem occasionally to miss a cycle only to resume normal periodicity thereafter.

3. Too frequent cycling

Some bitches cycle at 14–16 week intervals and are often considered to be infertile. This hypothesis is reasonable if the truncation of the cycle relates to omission of the luteal phase because of ovulatory failure.

A variant of this is the hitherto regular bitch coming into heat some 4–6 weeks earlier than anticipated, being normally attractive to males but in spite of being mated returning to pro-oestrus 6–8 weeks later for a normal, fertile oestrus. This sequence of events on an even shorter time-base has recently been observed in two bitches, both of which recommenced bleeding within 2 weeks of mating and one of which was successfully remated on the basis of vaginal cytological investigation which was suggestive of the normality of the second cycle of pro-oestrus and oestrus. This state of affairs would appear to be somewhat unusual but is a clear indication of the value of vaginal cytological investigation at least during the recurred cycle.

4. Anovular cycles

These can only be deduced to have occurred on the basis of circumstantial clinical evidence. Occasionally bitches which are normally sexually receptive show some resistance to mating and fail to conceive, but others show average libido. In the latter case it is possible that follicles have matured but not ruptured and such bitches should respond to injection of luteinizing hormone. It is best given within the 24 hours *prior* to mating in an attempt to ensure follicle rupture when viable sperm is in the reproductive tract; where several services at 24–28 hour intervals are envisaged the timing of the injection is not so critical.

5. Colourless or 'silent' heat

This occurs quite commonly but may only be noted by owners keeping a careful watch on the female genitalia. In such cases no observable pro-oestrus occurs. Signs include interest by experienced males, vulvovaginal swelling, a moistness of the vulva without overt discharge — if any discharge can be seen it is of a serous nature and may be colourless or at most pink-tinged. The bitch may show evidence of receptivity. In these cases oestrus is present as soon as signs are noted and mating should be attempted at once; service is usually achieved within 1–4 days of onset and is usually fertile.

Most breeders leave these bitches waiting for 'colour' to appear but the cycle lasts only 4–8 days and the bitch is into metoestrus before mating is attempted. Occasionally a slight blood discharge is shown at the end of such a cycle but by this time the bitch is no longer attractive or receptive.

6. Prolonged bleeding

Occasionally pro-oestral bleeding persists for an unduly long period, up to 6 weeks in extreme cases, and is often quite copious. It is assumed to be due to the failure of follicles to rupture and luteinize, but the administration of extract of corpus luteum or LH has given inconsistent results. In this context it is always necessary to consider the existence of pyometra or granulosa cell tumour.

7. *Nymphomania*

This is dealt with in Chapter 1.

8. *Increasingly feeble cycles*

These are mainly seen in bitches in which breeding has been deferred, often with the object of continuing a promising show career. Most affected bitches show cycles of apparently normal intensity up to the age of 2-3 years, but thereafter the oestrous cycle becomes briefer and with less obvious signs, e.g. vulvovaginal swelling is minimal or absent as are pro-oestral and oestral discharges. There is usually difficulty in getting these bitches mated, whether due to lack of male interest or non-receptiveness by the female. Usually affected bitches cease cycling completely at a relatively early age. Nonetheless on a few occasions, if mating can be achieved, a litter results and cycles usually return to normal. It is this syndrome which has led to the advice that breeding should take place at a reasonably early age if fertility is to be ensured.

Many of the above abnormalities, even if recognized as such, result in infertility, unduly long intervals between litters and the impossibility of planning a breeding programme.

Cystic endometrial hyperplasia and pyometra

It is difficult to imagine successful nidation on mucosal surfaces grossly changed as a result of the hormonal fluctuations of successive cycles. However, since the degree of change individually recorded is so variable and the condition is of such frequent occurrence, it is impossible categorically to state that reversion to normal function cannot occur. Indeed, as recorded (p. 16) successful medical treatment of open pyometra has been reportedly followed by fertile mating and pregnancy.

The extent to which undiagnosed endometrial changes of hormonal origin are responsible for bitch infertility is difficult to evaluate, and in the absence of more sophisticated techniques diagnosis must be made on the basis of direct examination of tissues.

Cyclic hyperplasia of vestibule and vagina ('vaginal prolapse')

This need not be incompatible with mating, conception and parturition but may, in extreme cases, present a barrier to intromission.

Failure of fertilization

Even following successful mating and tubal transit of spermatozoa, fertilization may not be assured. This may be due to hormonal, bio-chemical, antigenic or other factors not as yet understood.

Failure of nidation

Causes of failure at this level are not well understood but may be due to endometrial changes related to hormonal or other factors discussed elsewhere.

Fetal resorption

The extent to which this may be considered to be an aspect of infertility has already been discussed (p. 67). Factors responsible may, in the case of fetal overcrowding, be considered physiologically normal, whereas in circumstances of total resorption they may be thought pathological. Whether in the individual case the cause can be pinpointed is doubtful. In the case of repeated resorption by the same bitch to several sires, a basic hormonal or vascular deficiency may be assumed, although other factors, such as infection, cannot be ruled out. In the case of repeated resorption to a single sire, lethal genetic factors may be suspected.

Investigation will depend upon the initial establishment by palpation at 28 days of the existence of pregnancy. Thereafter serial serum hormone assays may establish premature withdrawal of hormonal support, although this facility is not routinely available. Microbiological investigation may also be performed.

An empirical treatment of this condition, which on purely clinical assessment is considered useful, is treatment with large doses of vitamin E. No explanation for the phenomenon can be offered, but it has been repeatedly observed that habitual resorbers may carry to term when so treated. Arbitrary doses of a minimum of 200 i.u. daily throughout pregnancy are suggested, commencing where possible some 2 weeks before the anticipated onset of oestrus.

Abortion

Although ultimately achieving the same effect, failure to produce whelps because of abortion need not necessarily be considered as infertility. However, habitual abortion may logically be investigated in the same manner as fetal resorption with consideration of lethal genetic factors, hormonal insufficiency, premature placental degeneration and/or chronic infection, especially by agents of the nature of *Br. canis* not yet endemic in the United Kingdom.

Infertility associated with infection

Venereal diseases

Although there is only limited recognition of venereally transmitted infection in the canine, interest in the subject is considerable. In areas of endemic *Br. canis* infection, where transmission may also be by contact with vaginal or fetal discharges, bitch infertility and subfertility are well documented. Bovine *Br. abortus* infection has also been hypothesized as a likely cause of bitch infertility, but this is unsubstantiated. Dog-pox lesions of the vagina and vestibule are not uncommon and seem likely only occasionally to present a barrier to intromission. Venereally transmitted tumours are rare and an unlikely cause of infertility in the apparently healthy bitch.

Bacterial endometritis

This well-established sequel to parturition may also be encountered in non-parous bitches. A wide range of bacteria is implicated and no individual bacterial species can be unequivocally indicted as the major cause. In case of suspicion of this disease as a cause of infertility, deep vaginal bacterial swabbing should be performed for isolation and sensitivity typing of the relevant organism. Prolonged systemic antibiotic therapy should be instituted, if necessary throughout an oestrous period.

Uterine lavage is not easily performed in the bitch, but in case of necessity good results may be achieved by instillation treatment of the anterior vagina.

Routine bacteriological examination of the uterus and anterior vagina in free-living street bitches has revealed a very low incidence of significant microbiological infection.

Bacterial vaginitis

Often asymptomatic, this condition involving a wide range of bacterial species is considered to be a major cause of bitch infertility. Systematic bacteriological swabbing of the anterior vagina by Hirsch and Wiger (1977) has confirmed the potential involvement of numerous bacterial species as well as their presence in many normal bitches, resulting in the statement that the significance of isolation in a particular case is probably directly proportional to the numbers of bacteria present. This opinion is further substantiated following the systematic isolation and successful treatment of a wide range of bacterial species from vaginae of bitches presenting infertility, often without obvious clinical symptoms of vaginitis. Infertility presumably relates to spermicidal factors, related to the biochemistry of bacterial growth.

Techniques of anterior vaginal swabbing are preferred because of the misleading picture which may present in the caudal vagina due to the passage of urine. To minimize contamination, eversion of the vulval lips is performed prior to insertion, when possible, of a sterile plastic tube as a speculum through which the microbiological swab can be inserted. To facilitate painless access to the anterior vagina the speculum should be inserted upwards along the posterior aspect of the ascending vagina then forwards towards the cingulum, avoiding painful probing of the clitoral fossa. In some cases vaginal diameter precludes insertion of a speculum and the bacteriological swab must be inserted alone. As control in such cases, preliminary swabbing of the vestibule and ascending vagina alone may be performed.

Vaginitis associated with cystitis

The aetiology of vaginal infection is sometimes obscure, but in many cases it is associated with previous or concurrent cystitis, often of a chronic nature, or with the presence on the same premises of a chronic cystitic. Because of this it is useful on initial investigation of an infertility case to include as routine a microbiological examination of a urine sample and to extend such investigation to include all kennel mates. In this way, hitherto unsuspected cases of chronic cystitis may often be encountered, especially in older bitches sometimes noted for their urinary frequency. The infections harboured and transmitted by these animals may be responsible for constant vaginal re-infection of otherwise successfully treated kennel mates, as well as for constant self re-infection. Logically, therefore, treatment of the cystitis should be undertaken, but in cases of extreme chronicity, especially with anaerobes, there may be only a very limited success rate and it may be wisest to consider isolation or culling of the subject to prevent total kennel involvement.

It is particularly difficult, even on the basis of serial sampling of the vagina and urine, to monitor progress in such cases and the rapidity of recurrence is sometimes suggestive of self re-infection from an unsampled site such as the urethra or clitoral fossa.

The precise mode of transmission between bitches is unclear, but presumably close bodily contact and the use of communal bedding and exercise runs as well as mutual and self-grooming activities play a part. These factors must contribute to the creation of a situation in which premises may be realistically described as 'dog sick', although such terminology is more often loosely applied to situations of general ill-thrift, subfertility and heavy puppy losses.

Unfortunately, in some circumstances, general systems of kennel hygiene employed appear reasonable and the situation appears attributable to simple overcrowding and in particular the use of communal bedding and small grass exercise runs as well as the opportunity for close bodily contact and normal social behaviour. In conditions of more obvious squalor regrettably prevailing in many overcrowded dog-breeding enterprises, and in particular the almost continuous use of whelping and puppy rearing facilities, disease transmission is more obviously understandable and the epithet more reasonably applicable.

In some bitches, the sudden recurrence of infection coincident with pro-oestrus after a period of apparent freedom from vaginitis is suggestive of descent of an intra-uterine infection.

Of particular relevance to the successful treatment of established cases of bacterial vaginitis, with or without concurrent cystitis, is tenacity of purpose, with repeated microbiological swabbing and especially sensitivity testing in order that appropriate adjustment in antibiotic administration may be made. It is therefore generally of little value to await the signs of pro-oestrus before sampling and contemplating institution of treatment, since in established cases protracted therapy may be indicated. Even in the event of failure to eliminate entirely an isolated infection, it may be possible to achieve conception by the administration of a prolonged course of antibiotic therapy commencing in early pro-oestrus and continuing through to nidation.

Of interest and relevance in this context is the observation of changing patterns of bacterial dominance. Thus, in cases of mixed infection, treatment instituted might successfully eliminate an organism of apparently major significance but facilitate, or at least fail to hinder, its replacement by the vigorous growth of an organism formerly noted to be present in relatively small numbers. By means of repeated swab evaluation, such changes can be noted and appropriately treated. Failure so to do might reasonably be assumed, in a proportion of cases, to invalidate the treatment applied.

MALE-RELATED INFERTILITY

Anatomical causes

Congenital lesions

Among the more obvious congenital lesions are those impeding intromission. In this category are relatively severe phimosis, persistence of penile frenulum and deformity of the penile bone. In cases of phimosis of a relatively minor degree, intromission may not be impaired although there may be difficulties with the tie and subsequent detumescence. Less obvious congenital lesions, possibly detectable by palpation, are aplasias of the epididymis and vas deferens, although in cases of a unilateral lesion fertility need not be impaired.

Acquired anatomical obstruction

Post-inflammatory stenosis or adhesions of the prepuce and fracture of the penile bone might impede intromission.

Postsurgical urethral stenosis and urethral compression by prostatic disease might possibly result in retrograde seminal emission, with ejaculation into the bladder, as recorded in man and other species. Conversely, postsurgical sinus drainage from the urethra will result in deposition of semen outside the bitch.

Acquired obstruction of the vas deferens may possibly occur as a sequel to prostatic disease, but is more likely to occur within the epididymis as a sequel to orchi-epididymitis. Failures to deposit spermatozoa due to such obstructions are deducible from the examination of semen samples obtained by manual stimulation and the examination of urine withdrawn by catheter.

Physiological infertility

The duration of spermatogenesis is species-variable as is the epididymal transit period necessary for maturation. For this reason, the degree of effect of transient physiological changes, even of a potentially damaging nature, is also species-variable. In general it appears that physiological changes, whether spontaneous or engineered by drug administration, must be of long duration before an appreciable effect upon fertility is observable, and it must be remembered that, according to the level of effect produced, infertility is apparent only after a latency of some duration.

Vascular disease

Effects entirely attributable to vascular damage occurring as a result of testicular trauma or inflammation are difficult to define. It has, however, been established that the disruption of sympathetic testicular innervation results in the degeneration of seminal epithelium and hypertrophy of interstitial cells, probably as a sequel to paralysis of the blood vessels.

Hyperthermia

The damage resulting from inflammation of peri-orchitis or orchi-epididymitis is variable and only partially attributable to hyperthermia. The meiotic phase of spermatogenesis is, however, particularly sensitive to chemical and heat damage, and it is probable that transient infertility following simple hyperthermia of the testes arises at this level.

Auto-immunity

As a result of acute testicular inflammation the integrity of seminiferous tubules may be broken down, exposing the immune system to spermatozoal (foreign) antigens and initiating humoral and cell-mediated responses constituting an auto-immune reaction to spermatozoa, spermatogenic cells and tubular basement membranes. Although the initiating inflammation might be unilateral, the auto-immune reaction is likely to be bilateral.

Hormonal factors

Hormonal control of spermatogenesis and the maturation of spermatozoa within the epididymis is complex and poorly understood (see p. 124 and

Prasad and Rajalakshmi, 1977). There may, therefore, be many factors, as yet unknown, which are capable of obstructing these normal physiological processes. Certain systems of male contraceptive control are based upon chemical interference with these fine hormonal systems.

Drugs administered intentionally or accidentally may act directly upon the cells of seminiferous tubules and epididymis affecting the production and maturation of spermatozoa, or they may act indirectly by interference with androgen production upon which both meiosis and the epididymal phase are dependent. The level of such interference with androgen production is also variable, being in some cases a direct effect on Leydig cells and in others an indirect effect brought about by central interference and the diminished release of LH.

Some of the commonly available hormonal preparations now widely used in clinical practice, as well as those hormones produced by pathological processes, can exert such damaging effects, but it must be emphasized that the degree of effect is both species- and individually variable, and much of the detailed information available has been obtained from studies in laboratory animals and men.

Some steroids can inhibit at pituitary level due to negative feedback systems. Testosterone itself may act thus, especially when dosed orally on a long-term basis as methyltestosterone.

Oestrogens also inhibit at pituitary level as well as directly depressing Leydig cell function. In cases of extreme exposure, regression of most testicular cellular elements may occur, except for spermatogonia and Sertoli cells, and recovery will occur only over a very protracted period. Progesterones, including medroxyprogesterone, will also cause suppression of sperm production after the initial production of abnormal sperm forms. However, there is evidence (Wright et al., 1979) that for the dog this may be a dose-related phenomenon, since continuous assessment over a 7 week period of dogs dosed by intramuscular depot injection with medroxyprogesterone acetate at 4 mg/kg confirmed no effect upon testicle size, semen quality or interest in oestrous bitches, although mean plasma testosterone levels were reduced by 58%.

These drugs will also, of course, tend to cause a state of reduced libido, as does the specific anti-androgen cyproterone which otherwise exerts its effects directly at the epididymal level, resulting in the production of immature, immotile spermatozoa. Other drugs effecting inhibition at pituitary level include reserpine, 5-hydroxytryptamine, iproniazide and methallibure, none of which is commonly encountered in the context of small-animal medicine but which may be met in pathological processes or in case of accidental administration of drugs intended for other use. In the same context, the effects of radiation, radiomimetic and nitro-aromatic drugs upon spermatogonia, and the effect of α-chlorhydrin and others upon epididymal tubular cells, may be rarely encountered.

Because of the apparently precise biochemical environment necessary for the imperfectly understood processes of maturation of spermatids, it is easy to appreciate that a wide range of chemicals in common usage may exert untoward effects upon male fertility. In practical terms, the production of abnormal sperm forms indicates malfunction at the testicular tubular level, while the production of formed but immature and immotile spermatozoa is suggestive of epididymal malfunction.

Accessory sex glands

The extent to which the secretions of the urethral glands and prostate may adversely affect the viability of spermatozoa is uncertain. It has been well established, by the successful use of only the second fraction of ejaculate for artificial insemination purposes, that their contribution to seminal fluid is not essential. In case of advanced prostatitis, seminal contamination with purulent discharge and blood may be anticipated to reduce fertility because of gross alteration of the biochemical environment and the known spermicidal effects of blood.

Karyotype

Chromosomal abnormalities, especially Kleinefelter's syndrome (the presence of at least two X chromosomes in the chromosome complement of an apparent male), are recognized in several species. In affected subjects spermatogenic function is reduced or absent. Definitive diagnosis depends upon examination of a karyotype of somatic cells or identification of sex chromatin bodies in cell nuclei. In the dog there is no distinctive phenotype analogous with the tortoise-shell or calico marking of 'male' cats.

Endocrine imbalance

There are insufficient data available on which to base assessment of measured blood levels of pituitary hormones in the dog. Measurement of thyroid hormone levels in some cases of reduced libido and reduced spermatogenesis, however, indicates the coexistence of hypothyroidism. Thyroxine replacement therapy may be markedly beneficial in some of these cases and may also occasionally improve libido in cases where measured deficiency is only regarded as marginal. Confusingly, in some cases of hypothyroidism libido remains normal, although there may be functional impotence and reduced spermatogenesis.

Psychological infertility

Problems associated with psychological factors may be largely overcome by correct management procedure, and infertility of this origin cannot be equated with infertility associated with organic disease of the reproductive organs. However, at the commencement of any investigation of male infertility and in the absence of positive evidence that ejaculation has occurred within the bitch, the possibility of failure to inseminate must be considered.

Deficient libido/psychological impotence

Affected animals may produce good-quality ejaculates by manual stimulation but fail to inseminate bitches, even when intromission has occurred. Many dog handlers mistake random thrusting movements for ejaculation and it may be impossible to ascertain whether or not a presumed non-tie mating has actually involved ejaculation within the bitch.

Excessive libido/premature ejaculation

The converse of the preceding situation involves the overkeen young dog which may ejaculate both first and second fractions prior to intromission.

INVESTIGATION OF INFERTILITY (Tables 5 and 6)

In a surprisingly large number of cases, at the time of initial presentation there is some doubt as to the unequivocal existence of an infertile status and on many occasions it is not immediately apparent whether failure relates to the dog, the bitch or both. Confusion arises in part because of the failure of many dog breeders to keep records of cyclic habits of individual bitches, and because of their frequent failure to accurately detect signs of pro-oestrus in some cases. Added to this is the tendency to mate all bitches on an arbitrarily selected day of the cycle.

Confusion relating to the male is often due to unnecessary secretiveness on the subject of his potency, and also to the surprising willingness of some novice bitch owners to accept the services of males selected by the stud owner and about which they know very little. A further source of confusion is the more understandable habit, in pursuit of specific blood lines, of coupling partners at extreme limits of the age range. This is usually the service, by an aged stud of uncertain fertility, of an untried maiden bitch, occasionally in several successive seasons because of initial failure. The use of untried young studs on geriatric bitches is less common since few breeders attempt to obtain litters from bitches beyond middle age.

Against this background, therefore, it s expedient not to accept at face value the apparent infertility of every subject presented for evaluation. Rather, it is preferable to re-assess each case hsitory prior to the commencement of physical examination procedures.

Table 5. Suggested routine for approach to an infertility problem on an individual basis

INDIVIDUAL BITCH

A.   **Breeding history**

I.   Has she ever bred and, if so, how many pups (a) born, (b) reared?

II.   On how many occasions has she been mated?

B.   **Reproductive cycle**

I.   Periodicity.

II.   Normality of each oestrous period as regards:

    a. Duration and extent of blood loss.
    b. Overt evidence of receptivity during oestrus.
    c. Apparent duration of oestrus as assessed by behaviour of bitch, male interest, vaginal smears.
    d. Any evidence of 'colourless' heats?

III. Occurrence of observable signs of false pregnancy.

C.   **Mating regime**

I.   Single or multiple service?
    If single
    a. Is day selected arbitrarily by owner because of custom or personal convenience, or is it selected by observation of bitch receptivity, male interest and/or vaginal smears?

D.   **Choice of stud dog**

I.   Is the male selected chosen for:
    a. Show-ring success
    b. Pedigree
    c. Known fertility
    d. Convenience
    e. Ability to sire good stock assessed on show quality?

II.   If the stud dog is owned outside the kennel is his history known
    a. As regards fertility
    b. As regards libido
    c. As regards frequency of use?

E.   **Health history of bitch**

I.   Has there been any illness, in particular any evidence of urinary tract problems, whether calculi or cystitis?

Table 5. cont.

INDIVIDUAL DOG

A.   **Breeding history**

I.   Fertility.
   a.   At what age was the dog first used?
   b.   Frequency of service? This should refer to the total number and frequency
      of services not the number of bitches. Rest periods, if any.
   c.   Average litter size. Is it within normal limits for the breed concerned?
   d.   Is the number of bitches missing increasing, and if so are these within the
      colony or visiting bitches from other kennels?
      This situation must be assessed in conjunction with the breeding history
      of the bitches which had infertile matings.

II.   Libido, bearing in mind both individual and breed variations, including age of
   sexual maturity. Has libido noticeably decreased?

Investigation and treatment of the bitch

Detailed preliminary history taking

This is essential in all cases. It is necessary at the outset to ascertain the age of onset of oestrous cyclic activity, regularity of cyclic habit and anoestrous interval; in addition, the normality of appearance of pro-oestrus and oestrus and the degree of presentation of false pregnancy symptoms following each cycle should be recorded. From this information, according to the breed of the subject, initial impressions can be formed of the normality or abnormality of signs presenting and of the likelihood of normal ovulatory cycles prior to breeding failure. History of any intercurrent or previous diseases, in particular cystitis and vaginitis, should also be obtained.

Details required of breeding failure include a full history of all breeding attempts, whether or not successful. In cases of occasional success it is necessary that the relationship of successful to unsuccessful matings be ascertained. The system of selection of mating day or days should be ascertained, as well as observations made of both the bitch's and dog's reaction at the time of mating. Details are also required of the fertility records of the males used. From this information it may be possible to form an opinion as to the nature of the problem and the likely direction of investigation in the individual case. In particular, it should at least be possible to ascertain whether intromission and insemination have occurred and whether or not the role of the male can be ruled out of further consideration. The breeding records of closely related bitches should be obtained if possible, and in the case of kennel bitches, the breeding and health records of all the bitch inmates should be obtained.

Table 6. Additional information required for infertility problems on a group basis

A.   Are both sexes involved in decreased fertility as assessed by the failure of visiting bitches to conceive?

B.   **Housing**

I.   Area available for the dogs.

II.   Number of dogs kept; this should preferably include fluctuation of numbers over a period of several years.

III. Kept in kennels with or without runs (*a*) individually, (*b*) in pens.

IV.   Are runs available to each individual or pair, or is a communal exercising area utilized and, if so, by how many dogs?

V.   Surface of runs with special reference to cleaning and disinfection and rest periods for grass areas.

VI.   Is a colony system of maintenance practised with groups of dogs running and living together?

C.   **Feeding**

I.   Quantity and quality with special reference to use of so-called complete diets with the protein content largely of non-animal origin.

II.   Any change in dietary regime which could be related to decreased fertility, bearing in mind that such effects may not be observed for at least 6–12 months after any change.

D.   **Breeding history as a whole**

I.   Are outside bitches conceiving to the kennel's stud dogs whilst bitches within the colony are missing?

II.   Is the strain mainly derived from lines of known good fertility?

E.   **Disease and vaccination history**

I.   With particular reference to any evidence of urinary tract infection in any of the dogs, including pensioners.

II.   History of pyometra in bitches of any age.

III. Evidence of recurring attacks of infection such as tonsillitis.

Procedures for investigation will follow logically from the results of the above history taking with priority given to:
    Routine clinical examination
    Attention to management
    Bacteriological investigation which should extend to dogs on the premises other than the individual(s) directly involved.

To some extent this information may indicate the likelihood of congenital defects and, more importantly, may uncover the hitherto unsuspected existence of a kennel rather than an individual problem.

Utilization of information

In some cases the information obtained is regrettably garbled and it is impossible to form even a provisional diagnosis, whereas in others the problems become relatively clear-cut. Thus, in a bitch of proven fertility, consideration of various congenital defects can immediately be eliminated and concentration focused on the likelihood of acquired disease or hormonal imbalances. Conversely, an unproven pet bitch living in isolation with novice owners will be considered a less likely subject for cystitis and vaginitis, and interest will be directed primarily to the establishment of normality of cyclic habits and in particular to the time of mating and the mating behaviour exhibited. Problems typically encountered in such circumstances are failure to detect true standing oestrus and bitch non-cooperation, either because of this or as a result of psychological disturbance and owner fixation.

Investigative procedures

The extent to which further examination and laboratory investigation are taken may vary according to conclusions already drawn, but in most cases it is worthwhile performing several of the most routine examinations. Thus, in all bitches which have missed after apparently normal mating, vaginal swabbing and microbiological examination of urine is worthwhile. In all bitches, especially those of unproved fertility, failure of males to penetrate and tie indicates the necessity for vaginal exploration at least digitally, but preferably also endoscopically.

In any case in which multiple mating has not been practised, or in which the male has exhibited relative indifference at the time of presentation, or in which oestrous cyclic patterns described are unusual, vaginal cytology should be examined throughout the following pro-oestrous and oestrous phases (*see* Chapter 4).

In cases in which ovulatory failure is suspected, either on the basis of vaginal cytological examination or because of the absence of evidence of false pregnancy in earlier cycles, serial hormone assay may be performed. This facility is, however, neither widely nor reliably available, and it is more realistic to suggest that after monitoring cyclic progress as described, ovulation be stimulated to coincide with mating by the systemic administration of LH.

In subjects suspected of resorptive infertility, serial hormone assay may also be performed, but within the limitations already described. In this situation and in cases of abortion, attempted hormone replacement therapy can also be monitored by serial hormone assay but this is difficult to effect without risk to fetuses and without risk of parturient failure.

In a number of cases the results of all examinations described may indicate apparent normality and it may be justified to proceed with more detailed examination. The limitations of soft-tissue contrast radiography in the bitch have already been mentioned (pp. 9, 12). Direct examination of uteri, oviducts and ovaries may in some cases be justified, especially in cases of suspicion of congenital defect or intersex status, but as stated, the evaluation of ovaries and oviducts by this means is difficult. At the same time, especially in older bitches with a history of obvious recurrent false pregnancy, uterine biopsy may usefully be performed.

Treatment

Various appropriate treatments of barriers to fertility have been mentioned throughout this book, and may be applied on an individual basis according to diagnosis. In cases of very minor structural defect, medical and even surgical intervention may be warranted, but in most cases cannot be justified. Thus a firmly rigid constrictor vestibuli (cingulum) which may be sufficiently painful to cause bitch resistance and to effect a barrier to the male, can in many cases be relaxed by low-dose chlorpromazine therapy to the bitch. In more extreme cases it may be ruptured digitally or surgically, and although this cannot be regarded as desirable, it is sufficiently close to the action of vigorous intromission by a keen stud to be acceptable. On the other hand, more extreme vaginal abnormalities such as the firm tissue bands described, if adequate to effect obstruction, should be recognized as abnormal and left untreated on eugenic grounds. Some structural variations, such as the sharply angulated so-called 'up and over' vagina, which are recognized by digital examination, require no treatment, as they pose little obstruction to experienced studs.

The value of multiple mating to a proven stud for as long as the bitch will stand, either with or without the benefit of vaginal cytological assessment, cannot be overstressed in the case of the healthy bitch for which no cause of failure other than mistimed mating can be established. The habit of routine administration of LH to such bitches is deprecated since its use implies innate hormone deficiency which should not be bred for.

Attempted hormonal and vitamin support of pregnancy is both difficult to evaluate and to condone, since it too encourages the use for breeding of hormonally inadequate stock.

Treatment of acquired disease, as stated, may necessitate a protracted period of drug administration. Certainly repeated microbiological assessment of the vagina and urine is indicated from the time of initial discovery, throughout the treatment period until pregnancy is successfully achieved. When indicated, rigorous medical treatment of cystitis must accompany the treatment of vaginitis. The use of systemic antibiotics is usually feasible, but in case of necessity, direct vaginal dressing can be simply effected via a flexible, lubricated polythene catheter.

Uterine lavage is not considered routinely feasible in the bitch, and in cases in which contrast medium has been forced under pressure into the vagina, there has been no radiographic evidence of leakage forwards through the cervix into the uterine body.

Investigation and treatment of the dog

History

As in the bitch, it is essential to obtain as detailed a clinical history as possible in order to differentiate the widely varying presenting symptoms. By this means it is immediately possible to differentiate the unproven dog from the mature animal which has suffered a sudden decline in fertility. It may also be possible to distinguish in the latter whether or not the reduction in fertility is relative or absolute.

In the case of the older dog it is particularly relevant to discover recent general health history and in both experienced and novice dogs the pattern of libido and mating behaviour should be established. In particular diminution of libido or expertise at stud work should be noted.

Utilization of clinical history

On the basis of such history it may be established whether or not the individual remains physiologically and physically competent to mate bitches. In affirmative cases, further investigation is directed towards the quality of the seminal ejaculate, and in the old dog offered at stud a routine annual assessment of semen quality is suggested. In cases of diminished libido, inability or reluctance to mate, endocrinological and physical factors require consideration.

In the young dog, psychological factors may also merit consideration. During such investigation it is frequently apparent that the dog handler has little appreciation of either psychological or physiological factors relevant to normal sexual function in the male (see p. 50), and it is often impossible to ascertain whether intromission has been effected and whether ejaculation has occurred. Such confusion may arise because it is widely known that the tie is not essential to fertile mating so that tumescence is mistakenly assumed to be inessential also.

Investigative procedures

In all cases a thorough superficial examination of external genitalia is relevant. In cases of apparently normal sexual activity but reduced fertility, this is unlikely to provide conclusive information, although signs of pain and swelling within the epididymis and testes, and in particular changed testicular consistency, may be noted.

In the subject which is interested but unwilling to consummate, or which withdraws in discomfort during intromission, this examination is particularly essential and lesions in and around the prepuce should be sought. In the case of the previously normal animal, traumatic lesions or dog-pox lesions may be noted, whereas in the novice dog congenital lesions such as restricted preputial aperture or persistent penile frenulum may be seen. In cases of diminished libido or non-arousal the general health status of the animal should be checked, with particular attention paid to symptoms of endocrinological disturbance, as evidenced by changes in skin and coat, weight gain, general demeanour and cardiovascular function. Such examination may reveal hitherto unsuspected hypothyroidism or even testicular neoplasia.

In cases of doubt as to competence of sexual performance, and in cases of normal sexual function without resultant conception, most dependence, following the basic clinical examination described, must be placed upon semen evaluation. The technique of semen collection by manipulation has been described (p. 58) and the value of the presence of an oestrous 'teaser' bitch discussed. In cases of reduced fertility which may be hypothesized to be due to diminished sperm output, it is particularly important that the 'teaser' be present in order to stimulate the production of maximum sperm output.

Evaluation of the ejaculate is on an empiric basis since information on this subject in the canine is limited. Traditionally evaluation is of the sperm-rich second fraction only, but in cases of suspected disease of the reproductive tract, especially of the prostate gland, a sample of third fraction should also be collected and examined for clarity and microbiology if necessary.

Evaluation of the sperm-rich fraction is on the basis of colour, opacity, motility and morphology, with only limited assessment of biochemistry and cytology. The colour is normally milky white or creamy. Yellow discoloration is usually due to urine contamination while red or green discoloration may be due to blood or pus. Opacity is proportional to sperm density and so a dense sample is desirable. The sperm count can be estimated spectrophotometrically or by Coulter counter if the instruments have been appropriately calibrated, but a haemocytometer is usually used. It is suggested that an average dog over 30 lb in weight probably produces 500 million spermatozoa per ejaculate and that ejaculation of less than 100 million may relate to subfertility, although less than 25 million may be required to fertilize. Evidence of seasonal variation of sperm concentration and sperm output recently published (Taha et al., 1981) suggests the months of March to June to be those of highest production in the south of England.

Motility and viability are estimated by examination of single drops of semen placed on a warmed slide beneath a warmed cover slip and maintained at approximately 37-38°C. Under these conditions good samples maintain motility for up to 30-45 minutes while poor samples may become inactive within very few minutes. Individual sperm motility appears relatively random, but a vigorous forwardly progressive movement of individual spermatozoa is considered ideal, whereas side-to-side movement without progression is considered unproductive. Taha et al. (1981) noted no seasonal variation in these parameters.

Smears stained with Papanicolaou or eosin-nigrosin dye combinations, or mounted in Indian ink, may be examined for morphology of spermatozoa and for the presence of blood corpuscles or foreign material. A higher number of abnormalities may be anticipated in the adolescent in which fertility is variable, but in the adult an incidence of morphological abnormality in excess of 40% is usually associated with low fertility. Abnormalities often encountered are marked deflection and sometimes coiling of the midpiece and tail. It is not, however, always certain to what extent some morphological defects may have arisen from preparatory techniques. Less ambiguous are symptoms of 'beading' of the midpiece and the occurrence of double heads or double tails. With experience, immature, primary spermatocytes may be recognized in some cases.

Biochemical examination is usually limited to measurement of pH which for the second fraction is usually between 6·1 and 6·6. Acidity tends to increase with keeping whereas, conversely, admixture with the third fraction will result in increased alkalinity.

In dogs used only infrequently, the first samples obtained may not be considered representative, in particular if a high proportion of dead or relatively immotile spermatozoa are noted.

Further examination may to some extent be dependent upon the results of semen evaluation. In cases of absence of spermatozoa, especially in young dogs, the presence of congenital obstruction of the duct systems may be suspected, but it will usually be necessary to repeat the sampling technique at least once to ensure that ejaculation actually occurs. This is detectable as pulsation by digital pressure in the region of the perineal urethra, and in the obstructed case there should at least be production of the clear first and third fractions.

In such confirmed cases of obstruction, further examination, though interesting, is unlikely to result in attainment of sexual potency and may, because of its surgical nature, be detrimental to the dog's subsequent show career. On these grounds investigation may be refused. Similar remarks apply to the proposed furtherance of investigation in cases producing damaged spermatozoa, since procedures will entail testicular biopsy which, because of the uncertainty of secondary effects, may be considered unnecessarily risky to a successful show dog. In particular the procedure is not recommended for normally fertile studs since such sequelae as inflammation, increased pressure, hyperthermia and induced immune reactions might seriously impair fertility.

Biopsy techniques are reviewed by Larsen (1977) who advocates the more controllable surgical method rather than various needle biopsy and aspiration methods. The surgical method suggested is to propel the testis forwards from the scrotum to the lateral penis in order to minimize the subsequent risk of adhesion between injured serosal surfaces. Through a small, longitudinal incision in the skin and serosa, the serosal surface of the testis can be exposed for selection of a site relatively free of major blood vessels. A small puncture incision of this surface may then result in bulging of testicular tissue which can be sliced off, or, if necessary, a fine, sharp blade may be used to scoop out a cone of tissue, although the risk of attendant haemorrhage is considerable. It is usually preferable to avoid suturing of the testicular serosa, but scrotal tissues may be applied with fine gut and routine skin sutures. Of particular importance is avoidance of tissue distortion by tearing or squeezing and the requirement for fine, sharp implements is stressed, as is the desirability of specific fixatives like Bouin's fluid, Stieve's fixative or Zenker formol rather than routine formol saline.

Further investigation of suspected auto-immune orchitis or of chromosomal abnormalities may be performed but not routinely. Tests for circulating antibodies against sperm antigens and for sensitized lymphocytes have yet to be developed in the dog, although these are used in man and experimental animals. Genetic investigation requires the employment of highly specialized techniques. Facilities for hormone assay are not readily available although accurate measurement techniques have been developed for some hormones. In fact, there is at present little information available relevant to the correlation of measured blood levels of LH and FSH and normal sexual function in the dog, and the quoted normal range of 0·5 to 5·0 ng/ml for testosterone apparently bears no correlation to libido. In fact, serial samples from the same dog exhibit wide variation within the range, while sexual performance remains relatively the same.

Treatment of male infertility

According to the outcome of the various investigative procedures described, precise diagnosis may be achieved in some cases and useful treatment effected.

In a limited number of cases, as described, psychological impotence or over-excitement and premature ejaculation may be recognized and treated, either with mild ataractic drugs or, preferably, with sympathetic encouragement and training. Acquired reluctance secondary to painful experiences or genital lesions may require a similar approach after suitable treatment of lesions.

In other cases the problem will be seen to relate entirely to the quality of ejaculate rather than to the sexual performance, and the prognosis will be more gravely in doubt. In the simplest of these the sperm content of ejaculate may be judged relatively normal and the prostate may be implicated as the source of contamination, either as blood or pus. Identification of the bacterial contaminant and its antibiotic sensitivity may allow successful if protracted medical therapy.

In most other cases the source of disease cannot be ascertained although it may be deduced. Thus, ejaculation of well-formed but immotile spermatozoa suggests failure at the epididymal level to effect maturity of the products of seminiferous tubules, while ejaculation of abnormal or reduced numbers of spermatozoa suggests disease at the level of the seminiferous tubule. Because of this imprecision of diagnosis, it has become accepted that the presenting condition, as appropriate, be termed idiopathic azoospermia or oligospermia.

Acquired azoospermia in the adult dog is relatively common and often associated with palpable alteration of testicular texture. In the majority of cases precise aetiology can only be hypothesized, but with increasing awareness of auto-immune disease mechanisms there is a tendency to implicate this as a probable cause. It is a matter for speculation whether initiating disease processes can be reliably attributed to relative overuse in youth, as is often suggested to be the case, although there is a considerable amount of circumstantial clinical evidence in support of this view. At the very least overuse of young dogs is to be deprecated from a management viewpoint in that reduction of libido and disinterest in stud work may often become apparent, although sometimes only transiently. Disturbance of testicular vascular supply, as demonstrated experimentally, and continuous exposure to female sex hormones may also result in azoospermia.

Azoospermia has not been found responsive to hormonal therapy other than the withdrawal of female sex hormones when these have been administered to suppress spermatogenesis.

Oligospermia has proved to be responsive to hormone therapy in man, using specific androgens — mesterolone and fluoxymesterone — which provide androgenic boost without negative feedback effect upon the pituitary production of FSH and LH, but their use in dogs is unreported. Most suggested therapies are too simplistically crude, being based on little understanding of the finer hormonal controlling mechanisms. A relatively logical treatment in the case of production of large numbers of abnormal sperm forms is enforced temporary suppression of spermatogenesis by prolonged administration of female sex hormones or anti-androgens. Following recovery from suppression, sperm quality may possibly be improved.

In the event of failure to effect improvement, fertilization may successfully be achieved by artificial insemination of pooled, stored ejaculate, although at the present time this is contrary to the rulings of the Kennel Club.

Regrettably, the treatment of infertility in the male is generally unrewarding in cases where sperm quality is adversely affected, except in cases where aetiology of the disease can be seen to relate to lesions in organs other than the testis and epididymis.

As a general observation, it seems that whereas formerly infertility was generally attributed to the bitch, there is now an increasing tendency towards the presentation of stud dogs for fertility assessment. It is unclear whether this indicates a trend of increasing male infertility problems or merely reflects an increasing awareness among stud dog owners.

REFERENCES

Doyle J. B. (1951) Exploratory culdotomy for observation of tubo-ovarian physiology at ovulation time. *Fertil. Steril.* 2, 475, 486.

Furneaux R. W. (1979) Surgical disorders of the canine vagina and vulva. *The Veterinary Annual*, 19th Issue (eds. Grunsell C. S. and Hill F. W. G.). John Wright & Sons Ltd, Bristol.

Hirsch D. C. and Wiger N. (1977) The bacterial flora of the normal canine vagina compared with that of vaginal exudates. *J. Small Anim. Pract.* 18, 25-30.

Holst P. A. and Phemister R. D. (1975) Temporal sequence of events in the estrous cycle of the bitch. *Am. J. Vet. Res.* 36, 705-706.

Holt P. E. and Sayle B. (1981) Congenital vestibulo-vaginal stenosis in the bitch. *J. Small Anim. Pract.* 22, 67-75.

Kessy B. M. and Noakes D. E. (1979) Determination of patency of Fallopian tubes in the cow by means of phenolsulphonphthalein and starch grain test. *Vet. Rec.* 105, 414-420.

Larsen R. E. (1977) Testicular biopsy in the dog. Symposium on reproductive problems. *Vet. Clin. North Am.* 7, 747-755.

Prasad M. R. N. and Rajalakshmi M. (1977) Recent advances in the control of male reproductive functions. *International Review of Physiology*, Vol. 13. *Reproductive Physiology II* (ed. Greep R. O.). Baltimore, University Park Press, pp. 153-199.

Sweeney W. J. (1958) Hysterosalpingography. *Obstet. Gynecol.* 11, 640-645.

Taha M. B., Naokes D. E. and Allen W. E. (1981) The effect of season of the year on the characteristics and composition of dog semen. *J. Small Anim. Pract.* 22, 177-184.

Wright P. J., Stelmasiak T., Black D. et al. (1979) Medroxy progesterone acetate and reproductive processes in male dogs. *Aust. Vet. J.* 55, 437-438.

FURTHER READING

Boucher J. H., Foote R. H. and Kirk R. W. (1958) The evaluation of semen quality in the dog and the effects of frequency of ejaculation upon semen quality, libido and depletion of sperm reserves. *Cornell Vet.* 48, 67-86.

James R. W., Heywood R. and Fowler D. J. (1979) Serial percutaneous testicular biopsy in the beagle dog. *J. Small Anim. Pract.* 20, 219-228.

James R. W., Heywood R. and Street A. E. (1979) Biochemical observations on beagle dog semen. *Vet. Rec.* 104, 480-482.

Taha M. B., Noakes D. E. and Allen W. E. (1981) The effects of some exogenous hormones on seminal characteristics, libido and peripheral plasma testosterone concentrations in the male beagle dog. *J. Small Anim. Pract.* 22, 589-595, 663-667.

Taha M. B., Noakes D. E. and Allen W. E. (1981) Some aspects of reproductive function in the male dog at puberty. *J. Small Anim. Pract.* 22, 663-667.

Chapter 13

Problems of Behaviour of Miscellaneous Origin

It is not uncommon for behavioural problems to occur which are related to the reproductive cycle in some way or another; these may result in actual clinical problems, e.g. during parturition, maternal behaviour affecting neonate puppies, or in behaviour patterns which make the dog less acceptable as a companion animal. Such problems may arise from fundamental temperament traits or may be due to faulty management by owners. The former is obviously more difficult to deal with and in certain instances, e.g. poor mothering performance, the trait should be bred out by eliminating bad mothers from breeding programmes.

THE BITCH

Physiological causes

Oestrous cycle

Few bitches show other than slight behavioural changes during pro-oestrus, these being generally limited to a changed urination pattern for 2-3 days prior to pro-oestrus and/or oestrus; this seldom causes any inconvenience.

The bitch is only sexually receptive during oestrus, a period of a few days, and even then may show little behavioural change. In bitches with a high libido constant efforts to escape and/or to 'call' to passing dogs may be very trying, especially as appetite may be decreased or even lost and the bitch unable to rest, thus presenting a somewhat distressing picture to the owner. Reassurance as to transience is usually all that is required.

False pregnancy

This has already been fully discussed (pp. 42–47) as a physiologically natural sequel to oestrus in the bitch, but in some cases may be legitimately regarded as pathological in clinical signs.

Bitches showing severe symptoms during false pregnancy become temporarily less acceptable pets whether due to sluggishness, psychological disturbance or lactation. When this period is added to the inconvenience of segregation during oestrus a bitch may be regarded as behaviourally abnormal for anyting up to 6 months of the year. Whilst the relatively transient inconvenience of 'heat' should be acceptable to anyone electing to keep a bitch, when this has added to it a severe false pregnancy, a quite significant problem can arise and it is quite understandable that owners seek professional assistance. Undoubtedly spaying is justified in such cases when it is clear that the condition recurs regularly.

Spaying

Spaying has become a very widespread practice with a considerable increase in demand for its performance. There has been a tendency to equate spaying in the dog and cat, whereas there are significant differences both as regards surgical technique and results. It is not proposed to deal with surgical technique in detail, since this has been discussed by Joshua (1965) and more recently by Pearson (1973) who has amplified discussion of the complications of ovarohysterectomy. However, it is considered worthwhile highlighting a few problem areas.

The indications for spaying, as distinct from that of convenience, have been mentioned under the various relevant headings as a therapeutic measure. In such cases ovarohysterectomy is to be highly recommended. However, it is becoming increasingly apparent that many owners of bitches are inadequately advised on the pros and cons of spaying, especially in relation to the complications listed. A surprising number state that in full knowledge of the facts they would never have requested that surgery be performed and would never, in future, do so.

It is true that in a modern, largely urban, society entire bitches cause considerable inconvenience but this is due to the lax control of the dog population. Were it to be illegal for dogs to be unattended off their owners' premises the problem would virtually vanish overnight. It is surely worthy of reflection that, with the exception of a small proportion of tom cats, the male dog is the only animal kept as a domestic pet that is allowed so much freedom in its entire state. Far too many owners of male dogs castigate bitch owners when it is their own management that is at fault.

It is suggested that the term spaying should be interpreted as ovaro-panhysterectomy unless discussion with the owner has indicated some reason for a partial technique, e.g. ovariectomy solely to prevent oestrous cycles or partial hysterectomy to prevent pregnancy, neither of which is to be recommended.

Due to the short ovarian ligaments and the fat bursa precise and complete removal of the ovaries is not always easy; the accurate laying of ligatures may be difficult and the ovary cannot be seen until it is extruded from its bursa. It is therefore very important that the removed genital tract should be carefully examined after operation to confirm that both ovaries have been completely excised. If there is any doubt owners should be warned accordingly, since even a remnant of ovarian tissue can result in continuing oestrous cycles which may be of irregular and frequent occurrence.

The dog is particularly prone to react adversely to buried ligature and/or suture material, especially if this is non-absorbable, often as a foreign body-type tissue reaction resulting in deposition of fibrous tissue around the ligature which may also be infected. Such reactions are seen both at the ovarian and vaginal sites. Clinical signs may be very delayed, up to as long as 2 years after the original surgery, thus the surgeon concerned may not even see this delayed complication.

Although these granulomas are not common they occur too regularly for complacency and when they do occur may cause exceedingly serious problems involving other organs. Removal of the granulomatous mass per se is not easy and when other organs are affected may necessitate such radical techniques as nephrectomy, enterectomy and partial cystectomy. It is thus essential that only top-quality absorbable ligature material should be used when spaying bitches.

Although the actual surgery is easier in prepubertal puppies it is now fairly generally accepted that spaying should be delayed until after at least one oestrous cycle. The following are some of the undesirable sequelae which may be minimized or avoided by refusing to spay immature puppies.

Body weight

Although increase in body weight is not invariable after spaying it is none-theless all too common. However, it is both less likely to develop and is often less severe in bitches spayed after maturity.

Persistence of an infantile-type vulva

This is less likely after the first heat period. Although such an under-developed vulva may not cause problems it can result in an extremely intractable perivulval dermatitis which causes clinical signs of a severity out of all proportion to its apparent seriousness; the condition is seldom easily treated and in extreme cases may cause the owner to request euthanasia.

Urinary incontinence

It is difficult to assess the incidence of this problem but it is undoubtedly of regular occurrence, mainly in bitches spayed as puppies. Administration of oestrogens controls the condition but undesirable side-effects often accompany their use.

Temperament

Although many owners would deny it — often they have no standards for comparison — it seems that many spayed bitches lack personality, some are frankly neurotic and, when spayed before maturity, they do not relate normally to other dogs of either sex, nor to their environment.

Management causes

Surprisingly often abnormal behaviour can be created when methods of management adopted by owners interfere with normal instinctive behaviour. Problems are more likely to arise in breeding establishments although they are by no means unknown in pet-owning households. Often the management is genuinely believed to be in the best interests of the bitch but in breeding kennels it may be designed for expediency, time-saving and in an attempt to rear the maximum number of puppies. In pet bitches which are unduly 'humanized' and which have not been encouraged to relate normally to other dogs even mating behaviour can be affected.

Parturient behaviour

The majority of bitches have inherited normal instincts but these can be modified either by sublimation, because of very close attachment to a human being, or by faulty management. When poor mothering behaviour is an inherited factor, as it is in some breeds which have a high proportion of bad mothers, it should be as rigorously eliminated from the strain as would be an undesirable breed characteristic as judged from the show viewpoint.

As indicated earlier (p. 72) first-stage labour can be unduly prolonged in pets which seek constant reassurance from their owners rather than seeking solitude as is more natural. Change of environment may also considerably retard progress and it is wise to discuss this aspect with owners when they indicate their intention to breed from pet bitches; all too often they realize too late that both the birth and the later presence of the puppies are likely to interfere with the normal running of the household and so be inconvenient. A pampered pet should not suddenly be consigned to an outbuilding when parturition is imminent.

In these respects breeders are less likely to create problems than pet owners although even removing a bitch from her normal kennel to whelping quarters may be unsettling unless she has been made accustomed to her new place very thoroughly.

Mothering behaviour

Most bitches have strong maternal instincts, and if they derive from a strain which is good in this respect, a satisfactory learned component will have been added during infancy. Normally a bitch will be very attentive to and defensive of her litter for several days after whelping and will only leave them briefly to urinate and defaecate. She should remain with her litter for a large part of the time for the first 2-3 weeks during which period, unless she is unusually thin-skinned and fine-coated or weather conditions are extreme, she should be perfectly capable of providing adequate warmth for her pups. Bitches which spend little time with their litter for at least the first 2 weeks of life are not good mothers.

In this respect the household pet is once again more likely to cause problems as many, after the first few days, show a desire to return to some extent to 'social' activities; yet, if they are good mothers, they do not want to leave their litters. A quite marked conflict between instinct and acquired behaviour can arise in this instance. With a degree of ingenuity it is often possible to arrange that the whelping box be so sited that the bitch can attend to both 'duties' without detriment to her litter. It is obviously undesirable that the pups should be subjected to undue disturbance but it is often wise to abandon the idea of quiet and solitude in a spare room and to compromise so that the bitch has easy access to both her litter and the other parts of the premises.

Artificial heat as a modifying factor in maternal behaviour

The comparatively recent work on hypothermia, especially that of Crighton (1968) focusing attention on hypothermia as a major cause of neonatal mortality in puppies, has resulted in an almost exaggerated response by breeders, often producing effects nearly as disastrous as cooling, by their recourse to the provision of artificial sources of heat in the immediate postnatal period.

Observation of bitches with good mothering behaviour demonstrates that warmth should be provided by *contact*, not radiation. Contact heat is derived from two sources, the very warm mammary area of the dam (analogous to the breast of a broody hen), the surface temperature of which is only very slightly below rectal temperature (Crighton, 1968), and the contact between individuals in the huddled group of puppies provided that the litter number is not unduly small. The normal mothering posture of the dam ensures that both sources of heat are available but anything which modifies this behaviour can result in harmful cooling.

Factors which modify behaviour include: uneasiness during whelping so that pups already born may be exposed to low temperatures during the birth of subsequent puppies; any abnormality arising during and immediately after whelping, e.g. metritis, lactation tetany; any undue disturbance which causes the bitch to become overanxious; lastly, the incorrect method of providing a heat source. Methods of dealing with the first three are self-evident but in the matter of provision of a heat source more veterinary advice is required.

Since most bitches can provide sufficient heat without any assistance this is to be encouraged whenever intercurrent disease, poor mothering, extremes of weather or an inadequate whelping place do not make some augmentation desirable. When provision of heat is judged necessary, remembering that contact is the natural heat source, it is logical that the artificial heat be made available in a similar way via whelping boxes with a heat source available in the floor as a low-voltage heated pad or blanket or hot-water bottles.

Crighton (1968) suggests a steady ambient temperature of 70 °F to be necessary to prevent hypothermia, thus avoiding the fluctuations inseparable from many methods of home heating, but many bitches, especially of the heavier-coated breeds, show discomfort at such temperatures if they are also in close contact with their litter. The result is that the bitch tends to move away from her puppies to cool down, thus leaving them for unnaturally long periods without body contact. This change in behaviour is most marked when the heat source is the much-loved infra-red lamp suspended over the whelping box. These lamps are therefore a quite unsatisfactory method of preventing hypothermia because of their effect on mothering behaviour. Far too many bitches nowadays spend too little time in close contact with their litters which is deleterious not only to the bitch concerned but, via the learned component of behaviour, to the subsequent behaviour of bitches from litters so reared.

To summarize, provided the mother's health is normal, a satisfactory temperature should be maintained by provision of a well-designed whelping box, no outside interference with normal behaviour and, if additional heat is required, it should be provided by contact not radiation.

Feeding the bitch during lactation

In the few days immediately following birth many bitches appreciate food being offered in such a way that they do not have to move away from their litter, a practice which facilitates good mothering behaviour. It is difficult to understand the popular idea that the bitch should be fed virtually as an invalid for 24–48 hours after whelping; it is true that some bitches do refuse solid food for a short time, but there is absolutely no need to impose a solely liquid diet. The bitch has expended considerable energy during labour, which, if uncomplicated, has been a perfectly normal physical activity and surely requires high-quality solid food to replace depleted reserves.

The very rapid weight gains of nursing puppies and the consequent stresses placed upon the metabolic processes of the bitch throughout lactation are discussed in Chapter 9 (p. 107).

Bearing in mind the relatively short alimentary tract of the dog, which is designed to deal with concentrated-type foods, it is clear that very generous feeding of lactating bitches is essential and that this should be in divided feeds, preferably 4 meals in 24 hours, to avoid overloading and discomfort. High-quality protein is essential as is a lavish supply of milk; most bitches take milk very readily after whelping even if they have refused it during pregnancy. Critics of this suggestion may point to the irregular food intake of wild canidae but, as judged by filmed records, the pups of such species can scarcely be considered examples of well-reared weanlings, and whilst it is undoubtedly true that a puppy in poor condition at weaning can make tremendous progress if the regime in its new home is good, the aim should surely be the production of puppies in first-class condition and which, in the majority of breeds, are self-supporting at 6 weeks of age. Possible exceptions are some toy breeds which may still be very immature at this age.

Artificial puppy-rearing systems

Artificial feeding is required for orphaned puppies, if the dam is unable for any reason to nurse them adequately or if the number is too large. In the last instance the wiser policy is to cull and reduce the litter to a number which can be coped with by the dam, but owners are often reluctant to adopt this practice. It is very important that all puppies should receive colostrum to ensure that they obtain adequate maternal antibodies. The subject of milk substitutes is dealt with in Chapter 9.

In the case of overlarge litters some breeders adopt the practice of supplementing the intake of all puppies of a litter on a rotational basis so that each gets some natural and some artificial milk. It is probably better to divide the litter so that some whelps are fed solely by the bitch and the remainder solely artificially fed to avoid undue stress on the infant digestive system of coping with two different milks, even if the composition differs only marginally. However, to minimize social disturbance it is desirable that all whelps lie with the bitch between feeds.

Although several techniques of feeding are available, including proprietary and contrived suckling devices, syringe feeders and stomach tubes, it is preferable that actual suckling be encouraged. The administration of measured volumes of feed by stomach tube is undeniably time-saving and in certain circumstances a useful nursing technique, but by deprivation of normal sucking is liable to result in extraordinary forms of suckling behaviour which may persist into adult life. The major precaution necessary in the construction of a teat is to ensure that the aperture is adequate to allow sucking without wind-sucking, but not so large that excessive volumes are taken in with the risk of inhalation.

It is also essential to ensure that the whelps get adequate limb exercise. Observation of normal litters demonstrates forcibly that the feeding behaviour of puppies involves considerable and vigorous use of both fore- and hindlimbs, the former during 'kneading' of the dam's mammae to stimulate let-down and the latter to maintain the pup in position at the chosen teat. It is perhaps not too fanciful to postulate that the absence of, or serious diminution of, this limb exercise could affect skeletal development both as regards muscles and joints.

Artificial feeding of puppies is time-consuming and demanding but if owners insist upon so doing it is the duty of the profession to advise them clearly of the problems. There is no short cut.

Advocated systems of maintenance of orphaned puppies, quite apart from those relating to feeding, are markedly different. It has been suggested (Sheffy, 1978) that the puppies should be kept individually isolated in separate compartments in order that weight gains, gastro-intestinal function, etc. can be more easily monitored and that problems associated with suckling of siblings can be avoided. This system, however, results in a state of almost total sensory deprivation, which seems both unnecessary and potentially damaging to social development; a system allowing full social contact with litter mates is preferable. Ideally the services of a foster mother can be used, for which purpose a lactating bitch in false pregnancy might be suitable, or failing this a non-lactating bitch with strong mothering instinct which is prepared to supervise the litter and attend to grooming, cleansing, etc. In the absence of so natural a system it is essential that at the time of artificial feeding attention also be paid to puppy defaecation and urination. This can be stimulated by wiping the anogenital region with damp cotton-wool pads. In the absence of a foster mother, it may also be beneficial to their social development to ensure that puppies are well handled at feeding time and not treated too clinically or in too dismissive a fashion. The provision of heat, as discussed, is ideally by an underblanket source and in the event that an overhead heat source is provided, attention must be paid to the risk of overheating and overdrying of puppies.

Puppies deprived of colostrum should be vaccinated at about 6 weeks of age since no interference with vaccine is anticipated in the absence of passively acquired antibodies.

Social development of puppies

Behaviour at later stages of rearing is important to the puppies in several ways, e.g. the learning of good mothering behaviour and socialization with both humans and litter mates.

Anything which causes the bitch discomfort will cause her to leave her pups more often than is desirable; sources of heat have already been mentioned. Damage to the mammary skin from the nails of the whelps is another, mainly seen at 3-4 weeks of lactation, and is often unrecognized by owners; it is dealt with on obvious lines.

From 4 weeks onwards the bitch will play with the offspring but is often deterred by their persistent and overvigorous efforts to suckle; the use of a 'weaning jacket' — the Baby-gro is a most useful garment — enables the bitch to play without constant molestation and appears to be much appreciated by her.

Socialization of puppies should be maximal between 4 and 7 weeks of age both as regards handling by humans and interaction within the species, the latter, whenever possible, can usefully include other adult dogs as well as puppies of similar age. If puppies are to become satisfactory and well-balanced domestic pets it is essential that they learn acceptable behaviour with other dogs as well as with humans, hence the importance of management at this stage.

Between 6 and 8 weeks of age is also considered the ideal time for transference of puppies from their breeder to their permanent home, coinciding as it does with the natural weaning, assertion of independence and formation of new social bonds outside the nest box. It is also the easy and natural time to enforce house-training habits as hard-feeding regimes are first established.

THE MALE DOG

Management

Most male dogs are not unduly highly sexed and can lead a celibate existence, apparently without problem, provided they are not exposed to oestrous bitches. However, many owners consult veterinary surgeons on sexual problems in their dogs.

Demonstrable sexual activity may be seen in puppies in the nest with pelvic thrusting and mounting attempts which are purely reflex and not dependent upon a sexual stimulus. Most male puppies show little sexual activity until puberty approaches, but occasionally puppies from 9 weeks onwards will grasp people's legs or other objects and make copulatory movements. It is important that this behaviour is vigorously discouraged and the offender be disciplined as with any other departure from acceptable behaviour such as absence of cleanliness in the house.

The period of adolescence is insufficiently considered in the context of management and veterinary advice. Not only is sexuality rapidly escalating but many dogs go through a period of 'teenage awkwardness' when they lose the dependence of puppyhood and to some extent become detached from their owners and generally less obedient. In some animals increasing libido results in quite unacceptable behaviour at which stage veterinary advice is sought, often with a request for castration. Whatever the pros and cons of castration it should not be easily resorted to at this stage. Adolescence is a transient phase lasting usually only a matter of weeks, but occasionally longer, following which the vast majority of dogs become perfectly acceptable socially and owners should be discouraged from a premature decision to castrate.

However, if treatment is required in such animals, the use of *very small* doses of oestrogen is usually very effective. The adolescent male is unusually sensitive to administration of oestrogens, hence the oral route is recommended at a dose rate of 0·25-1·0 mg daily; injections and implants should *not* be used. Bizarre and almost unbelievable changes may arise after implantation at this age, the tip of the penis sometimes becoming oedematous and vulval in shape and exuding a serosanguineous discharge visually similar to that of oestrus. Attractiveness to other males is another unwanted side-effect. In most cases treatment over a period of 4–8 weeks is adequate, preferably in interrupted courses of weekly duration. Total failure of response with persistence of unacceptable behaviour is obviously an indication for castration but this should be deferred for as long as possible and is only occasionally necessary.

Dogs not intended for a stud career, whether in a breeding establishment or as a household pet, should not be exposed to oestrous bitches. Pheromone attraction is often effective over quite considerable distances which does pose problems of management. One of the worst features of allowing dogs to roam unattended off their own premises is the inevitability of indirect contact with oestrous bitches, with the consequent disadvantages of sexual arousal in non-breeding males. All breeders who own stud dogs are only too familiar with the effect of oestrous bitches on males on the same premises, even if maintained in isolation some distance away. Most dogs become behaviourally disturbed, cannot sleep, often become anorexic and lose weight with startling rapidity. The exhibitor who tells a judge that a male exhibit is out of condition due to bitches on heat in the kennels is indeed likely to be telling the truth. Both dogs in regular stud work and those not so used are equally affected. Sedation is often called for in the interests of dog and owner alike. Drugs which have a pronounced effect on libido, e.g. potassium bromide, are more effective than ataractics or barbiturates.

The problem of managing young males later intended for stud work has been discussed under 'Mating' (Chapter 5).

Because of their anatomical make-up masturbation is not easy or frequent in the dog although full erection and ejaculation can follow copulatory behaviour with other males or inanimate objects, resulting in the familiar emergency calls to veterinary surgeons. Nocturnal emissions are likewise uncommon but do occur; Pekingese and Poodles have been most often represented in cases seen by the author. The typical history is of a dog found in its sleeping place in considerable discomfort, possibly with a wet bed. The discomfort is due to the fact that the penis is often not extruded from the sheath and has become engorged within the prepuce; this engorgement does not subside as quickly after ejaculation as in other circumstances. Curiously discomfort persists for several hours after detumescence, the dog having a somewhat arched back, stiff gait and being unwilling to move.

If repeated episodes occur, sedation, the use of oestrogen or castration is called for. Very careful history taking is required to elucidate the cause of the reported discomfort and may be difficult to obtain due to owner embarrassment; the actual signs are seldom present at the time of veterinary examination.

Physiological control of undesirable social and sexual behaviour in the male

Hypersexuality in the male may be defined as the manifestation of excessive or aberrant sexual behaviour. As stated, it is often arguable that problematical symptoms, however difficult to manage, are anything other than normal traits, since undoubtedly urbanization and systems of management employed may focus attention on antisocial habits which in the natural state or in the well-run kennel would be assumed normal.

Such symptoms include territory marking by urination, especially about the house, persistent mounting of other dogs, people or objects, excitability including excessive barking, gross destruction of household property, determined escape efforts, vagrancy (not invariably of sexual origin) and pack formation, and aggression towards people and other dogs, especially males.

Individuals presenting particular symptoms to excess naturally demand individual systems of management. Thus the sudden excessive destruction of household effects by previously placid individuals placed in an inter-male competitive situation may occasionally be controlled simply by confinement to robust kennels, though it is not unusual for other symptoms like excitability and excessive barking then to supervene, as well as overt symptoms of aggression. Whereas experienced dogkeepers, by themselves assuming the role of dominant pack leader, have demonstrably succeeded in running together large groups of mixed sexes and ages, it is often the case that this cannot be achieved and that the practicalities of each situation need to be individually assessed. It may therefore be advisable entirely to eliminate the competitive element by removal, or in some cases castration, of the less dominant dogs, whereas in other situations it may be possible to obtain temporarily beneficial effect without permanent loss of breeding potential by using specific antimale hormone therapy. As stated, this approach may be used equally well during awkward adolescent phases and to attempt control of relatively minor irritations like mounting, territory marking and overexcitability, but it is unfortunately probably true to say that the control of aggression is the least reliably effective use of these drugs, possibly because several factors combine in presentation of this facet of personality. In other contexts, anti-androgen therapy has been reported useful in achieving states of heightened receptivity in male dogs under training, whether or not previously exhibiting overt signs of aggression. It is assumed that in this situation the effect is due to a reduction of androgenic influence either directly or indirectly at the level of the cerebral cortex.

Although, as stated, low levels of oestrogens may be used for their anti-androgen effect, their long-term use is ruled out because of potentially damaging effects on growth and testicular function. More useful drugs are progestogens from among the range already discussed for use in oestrus control. These include oral preparations of megestrol acetate and oral and injectable preparations of delmadinone acetate. The precise modes of action of both drugs are unknown, but an antigonadotrophic effect at hypothalamic and pituitary levels is assumed, together with blocking effects at peripheral sites of androgen influence like the cerebral cortex and prostate gland.

Side-effects of increased appetite and lethargy are sometimes observed, but the efficacy of both treatments may be more difficult to assess on the basis of behavioural response, and it is recognized that individuals may be refractory to so subtle an approach to the control of entrenched behavioural characteristics. Repeat treatments at increased dose levels are advocated in cases of reasonable doubt, but even assuming this approach to behavioural control to be successful, its inevitable association with even transient periods of infertility militates against its use on active stud dogs.

Published dose recommendations for delmadinone acetate by the subcutaneous or intramuscular routes are somewhat arbitrarily gauged on the basis of weight, severity of presenting signs and previously observed sensitivity to the drug. Approximately 1·5-2·0 mg/kg is suggested up to 10 kg body weight, 1·0-1·5 mg/kg up to 20 kg and 1·0 mg/kg for heavier animals, though all doses may be safely exceeded since, in the event of a lack of response within 8 days, retreatment at the same or increased dose levels is advocated. In cases of favourable response repeat treatment may be indicated in 4 to 6 weeks although the duration of beneficial effect may be longer.

Megestrol acetate is administered orally at more variable dose levels according to effect. An initially high dose level of approximately 2 mg/kg for 7 days is recommended, followed in the successful case by 1·0 mg/kg daily for 14 days and thereafter at intervals according to effect. In refractory cases a doubling of the initial dosage is recommended for a 7-day period, after which, in the case of success, maintenance levels are suggested as above, whereas in the case of failure treatment is withdrawn. In successfully treated cases beneficial effects may continue for a considerable time after cessation of administration and from the experiments of Wright et al. (1979) it appears that at low dose levels neither fertility nor potential for arousal by an oestrous bitch need necessarily be impaired.

Neither the use of anti-androgen drugs nor sedatives can, on a long-term basis, suitably substitute for correct kennel management and control of individuals. Regrettably, in many multi-dog establishments such control is lacking, and it is not unusual for assorted males of little or no stud potential to be continually aggravated by a shifting population of pro-oestrous and oestrous females. Under such circumstances the need for retention of entirety must be considered in the case of each individual since castration, rather than chemical control, may evoke considerable temperamental improvement. Unfortunately, however, this cannot be reliably assumed since in some cases behavioural traits persist notwithstanding diminution of interest in bitches. In such cases, anti-androgen drugs can sometimes be usefully employed, presumably because of some direct action of these progestogens upon the cerebral cortex analogous to the 'calming' effects of progesterone.

Castration, rather than chemical control, should also be seriously considered in the case of individual adult pet dogs denied sexual expression and social contact but exhibiting symptoms of repression and frustration. Symptoms may include such masturbatory activity as already described, often with genital pruritus due to excessive grooming, hyperaesthia and a tendency to hysterical and aggressive behaviour. This syndrome, presenting particularly in hyperactive small breeds, is rapidly responsive to castration, and the changed demeanour, aided by increased appetite and weight gain, can produce a rapidly rewarding transformation.

Whether or not castration should be routinely recommended for individual male companion dogs remains debatable. Neither author favours the canine neuter, preferring the full expression of the characteristic differences of the entire animal of either sex. However, it has been persuasively argued that beyond maturity the entire, celibate dog accrues only problems from the continued production of sex hormones, with the tendency in later life for development of hormonally dependent anal adenomas and prostatic disease conditions as well as disease of the gonads themselves.

HERMAPHRODITISM/PSEUDO-HERMAPHRODITISM

These conditions may be clinically indistinguishable and it is probably true that a relatively large proportion of cases of both remain undetected throughout their lives. Both conditions are infertile.

The technical differentiation of the conditions lies in the possession by the true hermaphrodite of elements of both ovarian and testicular tissue, while the pseudo-hermaphrodite contains the gonadal tissue of one sex but the genital organs of the other. Some apparently cryptorchid males may therefore be presumed, in the absence of visible evidence to the contrary, to contain female gonadal tissue and some superficially normal females may contain male gonadal tissue.

In true hermaphrodites ovo-testes may exist unilaterally or bilaterally, or one side might be represented by ovarian and the other by testicular tissue which might descend to an extra-abdominal site.

In male pseudo-hermaphrodites the descent of testicular tissue in a subject presenting an otherwise relatively normal external female appearance may be the sole reason for placing gender definition in doubt. In other cases close and comparative examination will reveal the external 'female' genitalia to be of abnormal appearance and position, with the vulval lips sometimes set so low as to approximate to the position of the preputial opening. In most of these subjects the clitoris will be seen to be comparatively overdeveloped, containing palpable bony tissue. Growth of this clitoral tissue during 'oestrus' in the true hermaphrodite or at puberty in the male pseudo-hermaphrodite may occasion initial presentation for definition of gender. Thus apparent females are encountered having extra-abdominal testicular tissue and grossly enlarged and erectile clitoral tissue. Character change and temperamental uncertainty have been cited as associated features of the condition and evidence has also been presented of genetic aetiology in at least one breeding kennel. When siblings of affected subjects are examined, it is not unusual to discover comparable lesions among them, including varying degrees of vulval and clitoral abnormality in the 'females' and cryptorchidism in the 'males'.

Where relevant, treatment by surgical ovarohysterectomy and/or castration, together with the cosmetic removal of unsightly clitoral or malformed erectile tissue, is usually entirely satisfactory in the creation of the apparent neutered female. Most precise surgical attention must be directed to maintenance of urethral patency and this is best ensured by routine presurgical catheterization of the urethra. Following removal of relatively gross amounts of erectile tissue and penile bone a little difficulty may be experienced in the apposition of mucosal edges to achieve an aesthetically satisfactory result. However, in general this is eventually achieved by granulation, provided sufficient attention has been paid to the most advantageous placement of the urethral aperture.

REFERENCES

Crighton G. W. (1968) Thermal regulation of the new-born dog. *J. Small Anim. Pract.* 9, 463–472.

Joshua J. O. (1965) The spaying of bitches. *Vet. Rec.* 77, 642–647.

Pearson H. (1973) The complications of ovaro-hysterectomy in the bitch. *J. Small Anim. Pract.* 14, 257–266.

Sheffy B. E. (1978) Symposium on canine paediatrics. *Vet. Clin. North Am.* 8(1), 7–29.

Wright P. J., Stelmasiak T., Black D et al. (1979) Medroxyprogesterone acetate and reproductive processes in male dogs. *Aust. Vet. J.* 55, 437–438.

Index

abdominal distension in pyometra, 9
abortion, 67–8, 158
  due to infection, 68–9
  due to teratogens, 69–70
adenovirus infection in perinatal
  puppies, 114
adolescence in male dog, 185
agalactia
  mammary congestion misdiagnosed
    as, 105
agalactia mastitis, 105–6
anaemia due to post-oestral bleeding, 35
anasarca, 86
anoestrus, 29, 30
  clinical and practical aspects of, 33
  microscopical appearance of
    smears, 37
  prolonged, 155
anti-androgens in treatment of hypersexuality, 187–8
artificial insemination, 57–60
auto-immunity and male infertility, 162
azoospermia, 175
  following frequent service, 51

bacterial infection
  in endometritis, 159
  orchitis and, 130
  in perinatal puppies, 115–16
  in pyometra, 116
  in vaginitis, 159
behavioural problems (female), 177–85
  management causes, 180–5
  physiological causes, 177–80

behavioural problems (male), 185–9
  due to oestrus bitches, 186
  management of, 185–6
  physiological control of, 187–9
birth canal, size of, 78–9
bladder, haemorrhage from, 149
breeding, frequency of, 53
bromocriptine in treatment of false
  pregnancy, 46
Brucella abortus infection, 68–9
  infertility and, 159
Brucella canis infection
  infertility and, 158–9
  with orchitis, 130, 131
  in perinatal puppies, 115–16
BUN technique, 13

Caesarian hysterectomy, 101
Caesarian section, 93–101
  agalactia mastitis following, 105
  anaesthesia for, 95–7
  ethics of, 99–100
  following uterine inertia, 82, 84
  further breeding following, 100
  indications for, 94
  oversize fetus indicating, 85
  site of abdominal incision, 97–8
  timing of, 94–5
  versus assisted delivery per vaginam, 86
Caesarian whelps
  handling, 98–9
  introduction to dam, 99
  resuscitation of, 98–9
canine distemper in perinatal
  puppies, 114

191